100 HIIT Workouts

2019

N. Rey | darebee.com

First Printing, 2019.
ISBN 13: 978-1-84481-016-1
ISBN 10: 1-84481-016-X

Warning and Disclaimer
Although every precaution has been taken to verify the accuracy of the information contained herein,
the author and publisher assume no responsibility for any errors or omissions. No liability is assumed
for damage or injury that may result from the use of information contained within.

The Science Behind High Intensity Interval Training (HIIT) Workouts

High Intensity Interval Training (HIIT) is a short, intense burst of exercise, usually carried out over a period of time that ranges from one to three minutes with a recovery phase between repetitions. Because HIIT brings heart rate, aerobic and cardiovascular performance to near optimal levels it delivers impressive results in improvement in body fat levels, increased aerobic performance, increased metabolism, lower insulin resistance and improved handling of stress. [1]

HIIT also manages to provide the near perfect solution to those who have little time to exercise but still need to do something in order to maintain the physical fitness levels required for a healthy mind [2] and body. Indeed, it appears that the cerebrovascular benefits of HIIT make it a prime form of exercise for delaying the onset of ageing in the brain as well as the body. [3]

Brain Health and Mental Function

The research suggests that the high volume of blood flow, as well as the biochemical stress imposed by HIIT on the brain's signaling pathways induce adaptations in the brain that include:

• Increased neuroplasticity (the ability of the brain to form and reorganize synaptic connections)
• Higher dendritic density (an increase in the brain's signaling pathways)
• Greater neuronal mass (the number of neurons in the brain)
• Better cognitive functioning (the ability of the brain to recruit one or more brain regions in coherent, analytical thought affecting learning, memory and decision making)
• Improved neurovascular coupling (the relationship between local neural activity and subsequent changes in cerebral blood flow)
• Improved angiogenesis (the development of new blood vessels)
• Reduced inflammation
• Reduced arterial stiffness
• Greater metabolic control

Brain health is a key component in delivering a better quality of life as we age. Exercise that benefits us in this specific area decreases the likelihood of reduced function due to ageing or crippling disease.

Stronger and Fitter in Less Time
Recent research carried out the University of British Columbia at Okanagan [4] demonstrates that the physical benefits of HIIT workouts versus continuous moderate-intensity exercise that requires longer times and greater frequency are:

• Increase in explosiveness, speed and agility [5]
• Improved cardiovascular health
• Increase in peak power output [6]
• Higher aerobic performance
• Better metabolic capacity
• Faster fat reduction [7]
• Greater endurance [8]

There is even evidence that HIIT helps combat and reverse type 2 diabetes [9] and can deliver significant health benefits to people suffering from obesity or cardiovascular disorders and increases muscle density in those who engage in it across all age groups and physical levels of fitness [10, 11].

The mechanism through which HIIT training delivers such powerful results for such small investment in training time was discovered in a study undertaken by principal investigator Håkan Westerblad, professor at Karolinska Institutet's Department of Physiology and Pharmacology which took muscle biopsies after HIIT sessions. The biopsies showed significant disruption in the calcium channels of individual cells within the muscle. [12, 13]. Calcium channel disruption triggers strong adaptive response in individual cells and encourages the production of mitochondria that act as power plants within a cell. HIIT therefore causes adaptive changes at a cellular level that improve fuel efficiency and power output of muscle fibers.

HIIT: How Often and at What Age?
This begs the question: are there limitations in the number of times we could do HIIT and are there age restrictions that apply? Research carried out by the Department of Life and Health Sciences at the University of Nicosia, Cyprus and the School of Physical Education and Sports Science, National and Kapodistrian University of Athens, Greece indicates that three to four times a week is the maximum beneficial number of times HIIT should be engaged in for maximal results [14].

The reason for this lies in the mechanical damage suffered by the muscles during HIIT work which requires adequate rest in order to recover and improve performance. The recovery period will have to be adapted to each person's recovery speed which differs according to a wide range of factors that include diet, medical history, sex and fitness level so it's worth experimenting with frequency until you find what works best for you. That means that you might have to go down in the number of HIIT sessions per week but it is highly unlikely that you will go up.

Are there any age restrictions when it comes to HIIT?

A Mayo Clinic study that looked at changes to the skeletal muscles at a cellular level [15] found that HIIT benefits individuals at any age and there is no upper limit that would stop people from doing it. The study revealed that HIIT may help reverse some of the ageing process by increasing the capacity of cells to express very specific genes as a result of adaptations they undergo because of the intensity of the HIIT workout.

When it comes to placing a lower age limit a recent study carried out Dr David Moreau, at the University of Auckland in New Zealand looked at the effects of HIIT on 318 young children between 7 and 13 years. The findings showed that in addition to the expected beneficial changes in cardiovascular fitness and strength, there were significant cognitive improvements experienced by all the children. [17]

In addition, other studies have shown that short bouts of exercise alleviate some of the difficulties typically associated with Attention-deficit/hyperactivity disorder (ADHD) in children. The only stipulation for young children is that the HIIT session is between ten and twenty minutes long to account for their age.

Summary
HIIT training resets the body and mind, turning back the clock for older participants and significantly boosting the performance of both mind and body for younger ones. As with all forms of exercise it is best when it is tailored to age and ability to help reach and overcome existing limits without running the risk of exhaustion or overtraining.

1.	Boutcher SH. High-intensity intermittent exercise and fat loss. J Obes. 2010; 2011:868305.

2.	Jiménez-Maldonado A, Rentería I, García-Suárez PC, Moncada-Jiménez J, Freire-Royes LF. The Impact of High-Intensity Interval Training on Brain Derived Neurotrophic Factor in Brain: A Mini-Review. Front Neurosci. 2018;12:839. Published 2018 Nov 14. doi:10.3389/fnins. 2018.00839

3.	Lucas SJ, Cotter JD, Brassard P, Bailey DM. High-intensity interval exercise and cerebrovascular health: curiosity, cause, and consequence. J Cereb Blood Flow Metab. 2015;35(6):902-11.

4.	Kilpatrick, Marcus & Jung, Mary & Little, Jonathan. (2014). High-intensity interval training: A review of physiological and psychological responses. ACSM's Health and Fitness Journal. 18. 11-16. 10.1249/FIT.0000000000000067.

5.	TY - JOUR DO - 10.1088/1742-6596/947/1/012045, UR - http://dx.doi. org/10.1088/1742-6596/947/1/012045, TI - Effects of High Intensity Interval Training on Increasing Explosive Power, Speed, and Agility, T2 - Journal of Physics: Conference Series,

6.	Herbert P, Hayes LD, Sculthorpe NF, Grace FM. HIIT produces increases in muscle power and free testosterone in male masters athletes. Endocr Connect. 2017;6(7):430-436.

7.	Shiraev, Timothy & Barclay, Gabriella. (2012). Evidence based exercise: Clinical benefits of high intensity interval training. Australian family physician. 41. 960-2.

8.	Gillen JB, Percival ME, Skelly LE, Martin BJ, Tan RB, Tarnopolsky MA, et al. (2014) Three Minutes of All-Out Intermittent Exercise per Week Increases Skeletal Muscle Oxidative Capacity and Improves Cardiometabolic Health. PLoS ONE 9(11): e111489. https://doi. org/10.1371/journal.pone.0111489

9.	The effects of free-living interval-walking training on glycemic control, body composition, and physical fitness in type 2 diabetic patients: a randomized, controlled trial. Karstoft, Kristian, Centre of Inflammation and Metabolism, Department of Infectious Diseases and CMRC, Rigshospitalet, Faculty of Health Sciences, University of Copenhagen, Copenhagen, Denmark.

10.	Sprint interval and endurance training are equally effective in increasing muscle microvascular density and eNOS content in sedentary males. 641-56, 10.1113/ jphysiol.2012.239566 [doi] Cocks, Matthew, Exercise Metabolism Research Group, School of Sport and Exercise Sciences, University of Birmingham, Edgbaston, Birmingham B15 2TT, UK. The Journal of physiology, J Physiol. 2013 Feb 1;591(3):603-4. PMID: 23378422.

11.	Comparison of Responses to Two High-Intensity Intermittent Exercise Protocols https://journals.lww.com/nsca- jscr/Fulltext/2014/11000/Comparison_of_Responses_to_ Two_High_Intensity.3.aspx, Gist, NH, Freese, EC, and Cureton, KJ. J Strength Cond Res 28(11): 3033–3040.

12.	Ryanodine receptor fragmentation and sarcoplasmic reticulum leak after one session of high-intensity interval exercise. Proceedings of the National Academy of Sciences, 15492, 15497, 10.1073/pnas.1507176112. Vol. 112. Place, Nicolas, Ivarsson, Niklas, Venckunas, Tomas, Neyroud, Daria, Brazaitis, Marius, Cheng, Arthur J. 2015/12/15.

13.	Intensity matters: Ryanodine receptor regulation during exercise. Tobias Kohl, Gunnar Weninger, Ran Zalk, Philip Eaton, and Stephan E. Lehnart. PNAS December 15, 2015 112 (50) 15271-15272; published ahead of print December 2, 2015 https://doi.org/10.1073/ pnas.1521051112

14.	High-intensity Interval Training Frequency: Cardiometabolic Effects and Quality of Life, 210-217. 10.1055/s-0043-125074 [doi], Georg Thieme Verlag KG Stuttgart. New York. Stavrinou, Pinelopi S, Department of Life and Health Sciences, University of Nicosia, Nicosia, Cyprus. Bogdanis, Gregory C, School of Physical Education and Sports Science, National and Kapodistrian University of Athens, Athens, Greece. Int J Sports Med. 2018 Feb.

15.	Enhanced Protein Translation Underlies Improved Metabolic and Physical Adaptations to Different Exercise Training Modes in Young and Old Humans. Matthew M. Robinson,

Surendra Dasari, Adam R. Konopka, Rickey E. Carter, Ian R. Lanza, K. Sreekumaran Nair 3. Published: March 7, 2017. DOI:https://doi.org/10.1016/j.cmet.2017.02.009

16.   Eddolls WTB, McNarry MA, Stratton G, Winn CON, Mackintosh KA. High-Intensity Interval Training Interventions in Children and Adolescents: A Systematic Review. Sports Med. 2017;47(11):2363-2374.

17.   Moreau D, Kirk IJ, Waldie KE. High-intensity training enhances executive function in children in a randomized, placebo-controlled trial. Elife. 2017;6:e25062. Published 2017 Aug 22. doi:10.7554/eLife.25062

100 HIIT workouts

1. Action Time
2. Activator
3. Adrenaline Rush
4. Ants in My Pants
5. Beginner HIIT
6. Belly Burner
7. Better Tomorrow
8. Blaster
9. Blueprint
10. Boiler Room
11. Boxer
12. Bulletproof Abs
13. Burn Mode
14. Burn Zone
15. Cardio Dive
16. Cardio Mixer
17. Cardio Prime
18. Cardio Pro
19. Carpe Diem
20. Catch
21. Chisel Express
22. Chopper
23. Coda
24. Combat Burpee
25. Confessor
26. Core Burn
27. Core Sculpt
28. Crossfire
29. Cursor
30. Double Helix
31. Drifter
32. Expedited Delivery
33. Fab Abs
34. Fast & Dangerous
35. Fire Punch
36. Flamethrower
37. Flyby
38. Free Fall
39. Game Changer
40. Genesis
41. Get It Done
42. Grasshopper
43. Grind
44. Hear Me Roar
45. Hell's Circuit
46. Heyday
47. Homemade Hero
48. Hotfoot
49. Howler
50. Huff & Puff
51. Incinerator
52. Inferno
53. Intervention
54. Into The Fire
55. Mass Blast
56. Max Impact
57. Max Out
58. Melt Off
59. New Beginning
60. No One Is Watching
61. No Surrender
62. Odyssey
63. Out Of Excuses
64. Overdrive
65. Overhaul
66. Over The Rainbow
67. Persephone
68. Phoenix Burn
69. Pouncer
70. Power Bolt
71. Power Melt
72. Power Shed
73. Power Strike
74. Power Trim
75. Purge
76. Quick HIIT
77. Rambler
78. Rapid Fire
79. Reanimator
80. Recalibrator
81. Reckoning
82. Rectifier
83. Refiner
84. Respawn
85. Reviver
86. Rewired
87. Ricochet
88. Rocket Fuel
89. Run & Gun
90. Scissors
91. Shifter
92. Silver
93. Sizzler
94. Skydiver
95. Smoking Hot
96. SOS
97. Super Burn
98. Super HIIT
99. Sweat Inc.
100. Toaster

Introduction

Bodyweight training may look easy, but if you are not used to it, it's very far from that. It is just as intense as running and it is just as challenging so if you struggle with it at the very beginning, it's perfectly ok — you will get better at it once you start doing it regularly. Do it at your own pace and take longer breaks if you need to.

You can start with a single individual workout from the collection and see how you feel. If you are new to bodyweight training always start any workout on Level I (level of difficulty).

You can pick any number of workouts per week, usually between 3 and 5 and rotate them for maximum results.

Some workouts are more suitable for weight loss and toning up and others are more strength oriented, some do both. To make it easier for you to choose, they have all been labelled according to FOCUS, use it to design a training regimen based on your goal.

High Burn and Strength oriented workouts will help you with your weight, aerobic capacity and muscle tone, some are just more specialized, but it doesn't mean you should exclusively focus on one or the other. Whatever your goal with bodyweight training you'll benefit from doing exercises that produce results in both areas.

This collection has been designed to be completely no-equipment for maximum accessibility so several bodyweight exercises like pull-ups have been excluded. If you want to work on your biceps and back more and you have access to a pull-up bar, have one at home or can use it somewhere else like the nearest playground (monkey bars), you can do wide and close grip pull-ups, 3 sets to failure 2-3 times a week with up to 2 minutes rest in between sets in addition to your training. Alternatively, you can add pull-ups at the beginning or at the end of every set of a Strength Oriented workout.

All of the routines in this collection are suitable for both men and women, no age restrictions apply.

The Manual

Workout posters are read from left to right and contain the following information: grid with exercises (images), amount of time to perform it for next to each, number of sets for your fitness level (I, II or III) and rest time.

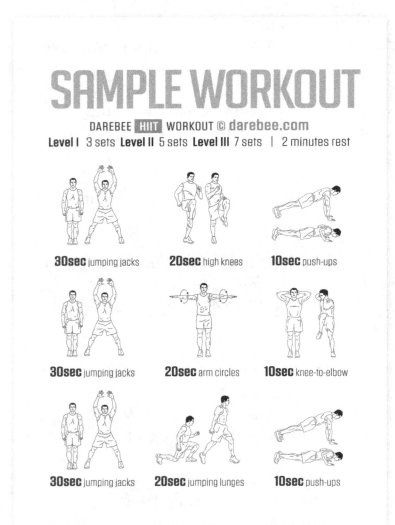

Difficulty Levels:

Level I: normal

Level II: hard

Level III: advanced

1 set

30 seconds jumping jacks

20 seconds high knees

10 seconds push-ups

30 seconds jumping jacks

20 seconds arm circles

10 seconds knee-to-elbow

30 seconds jumping jacks

20 seconds jumping lunges

10 seconds push-ups

Up to 2 minutes rest between sets

30 seconds, 60 seconds or 2 minutes - it's up to you.

All workouts in this collection are time-based. You will need a stopwatch to keep the intervals. Get a stopwatch or download a stopwatch app on your mobile phone. Alternatively, go to darebee.com/filter, find the workout you want to do and use an on-page timer.

The transition from exercise to exercise is an important part of each circuit (set) - it is often what makes a particular workout more effective.

Transitions are carefully worked out to hyperload specific muscle groups more for better results. For example if you see a plank followed by push-ups it means that you start performing push-ups right after you finished with the plank avoiding dropping your body on the floor in between.

There is no rest between exercises - only after sets, unless specified otherwise. You have to complete the entire set going from one exercise to the next as fast as you can before you can rest.

What does "up to 2 minutes rest" mean: it means you can rest for up to 2 minutes but the sooner you can go again the better. Eventually your recovery time will improve naturally, you won't need all two minutes to recover - and that will also be an indication of your improving fitness.

Recommended rest time:

Level I: 2 minutes or less
Level II: 60 seconds or less
Level III: 30 seconds or less

If you can't do all out push-ups yet on Level I it is perfectly acceptable to do knee push-ups instead. The modification works the same muscles as a full push-up but lowers the load significantly helping you build up on it first. It is also ok to switch to knee push-ups at any point if you can no longer do full push-ups in the following sets.

EC stands for "Extra Credit".

Video Exercise Library
http://darebee.com/video

The workouts are organized in alphabetical order so you can find the workouts you favor easier and faster.

1 Action Time

Action Time Workout is, essentially, a supercharged burpee but with double the pain you get double the benefits. Keep your body straight during planks and don't drop down during planks and their transitions. Your ultimate goal is to keep the plank throughout never dropping down to your knees... even though you will really, really want to.

Extra Credit: Keep the plank throughout the set.

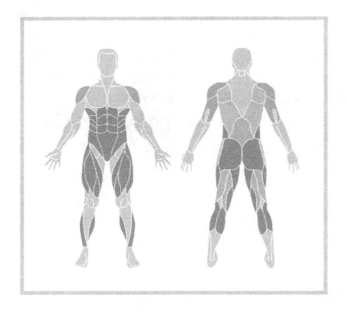

Difficulty

ACTION TIME

DAREBEE `HIIT` WORKOUT © darebee.com

Level I 3 sets **Level II** 5 sets **Level III** 7 sets | 2 minutes rest

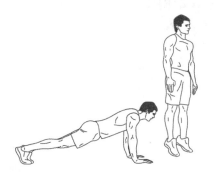

20sec basic burpees

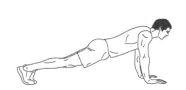

20sec plank hold

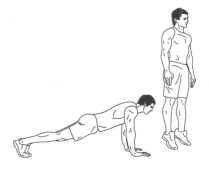

20sec basic burpees

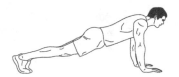

20sec plank hold

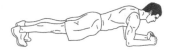

20sec elbow plank hold

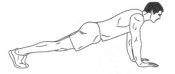

20sec plank hold

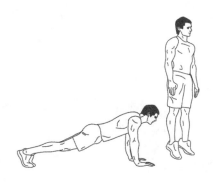

20sec basic burpees

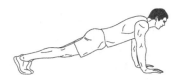

20sec plank hold

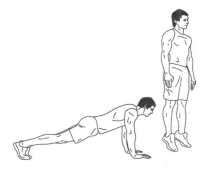

20sec basic burpees

2 Activator

Get your body moving and challenge your fascial fitness with an HIIT workout that requires you to move in a truly coordinated, balanced way. You work everything here and the load piles up as the workout progresses. Add EC for that extra edge and what you have is a workout that keeps on challenging you with every set you do.

Extra Credit: 1 minute rest between sets.

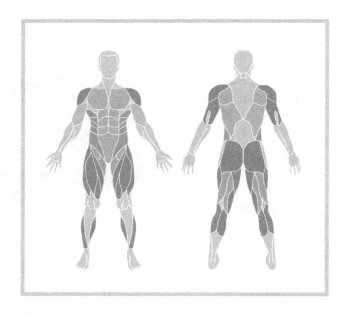

Difficulty

activator

DAREBEE HIIT WORKOUT © darebee.com

LEVEL I 3 sets **LEVEL II** 5 sets **LEVEL III** 7 sets **REST** up to 2 minutes

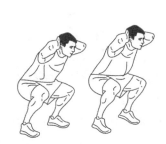

15sec squat hops

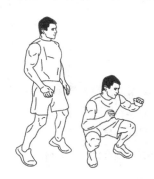

15sec bounce + squat

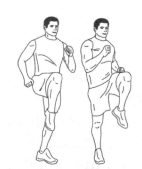

15sec high knees

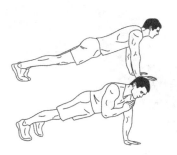

15sec shoulder taps

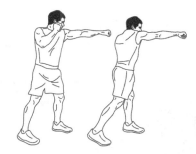

15sec punches

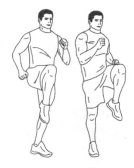

15sec high knees

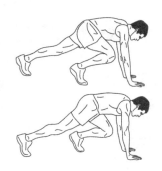

15sec climbers

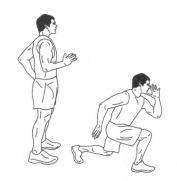

15sec sprinter lunges

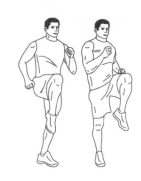

15sec high knees

3   **Adrenaline Rush**

Adrenaline Rush is a fast-paced, High Intensity Interval training Workout that loads the body's major muscle groups quickly, raises body temperature and pushes your body's performance to the max. This is a level four workout so you'll get into the sweat zone pretty much from the first set. The load to your lungs is going to be significant as the body's major muscle groups are challenged, but by leaving almost no muscle group untargeted this is the kind of workout you go to when you are looking for something that will seriously challenge your fitness and sculpt your body. Do everything as fast as possible, trying to up the rep count and focus on the EC for added difficulty.

Extra Credit: Hit the same number of push-ups every time.

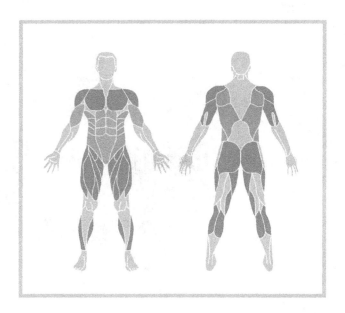

Difficulty

ADRENALINE RUSH

DAREBEE HIIT WORKOUT
© darebee.com
Level I 3 sets **Level II** 5 sets **Level III** 7 sets
up to 2 minutes rest between sets

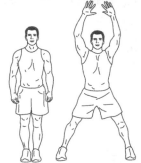

15sec jumping jacks

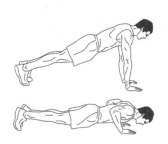

15sec push-ups

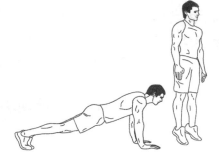

15sec basic burpees

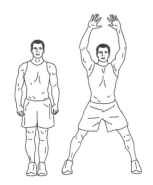

15sec jumping jacks

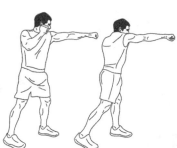

15sec punches

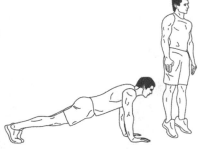

15sec basic burpees

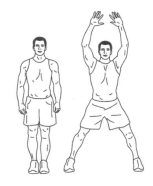

15sec jumping jacks

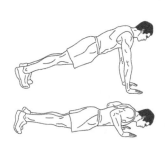

15sec push-ups

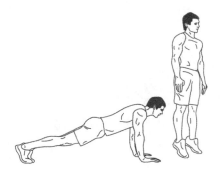

15sec basic burpees

4   Ants in My Pants

Ants In My Pants lives up to its billing because you literally have zero downtime here. With exercises that flow from standing up to floor and back the workout uses Jumping Jacks to jack-up the pressure pushing not just your calf muscles to the limit but also your VO2 Max. Remember your heels never touch down during Jumping Jacks and your fingertips meet at the apex point over your head. Master it!

Extra Credit: Hit the same number of burpees each time.

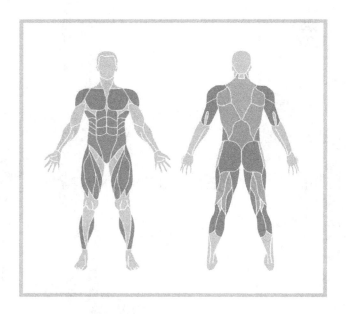

Difficulty

Ants in My Pants

DAREBEE HIIT WORKOUT © darebee.com

Level I 3 sets **Level II** 5 sets **Level III** 7 sets | 2 minutes rest

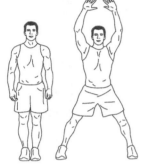

20sec jumping jacks

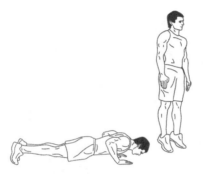

20sec burpees

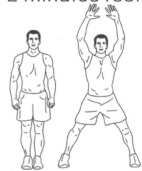

20sec jumping jacks

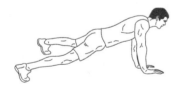

20sec wide plank hold

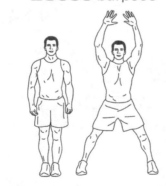

20sec jumping jacks

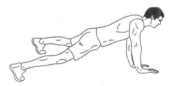

20sec wide plank hold

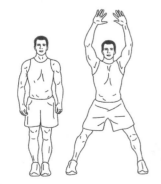

20sec jumping jacks

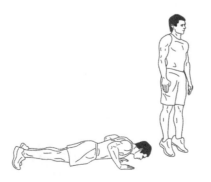

20sec burpees

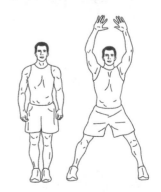

20sec jumping jacks

5 Beginner HIIT

The Beginner HIIT Workout is perfect if you are running low on energy, short on time or if you are just starting out with HIIT. It's not hard yet it is demanding enough to give you a good burn. Try to go flat out each time - after all, it's only 15 seconds. You can do anything for 15 seconds!

Extra Credit: 1 minute rest between sets.

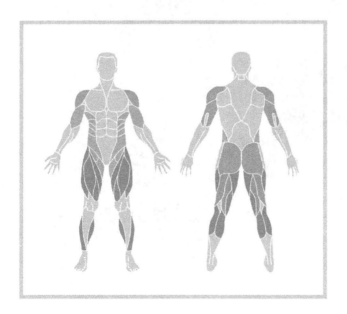

Difficulty

Beginner
HIIT

DAREBEE WORKOUT
© darebee.com
repeat 5 times in total
up to 2 minutes rest between sets

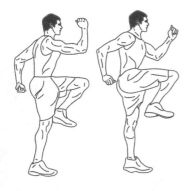

15sec march steps

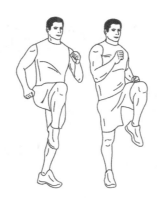

15sec high knees

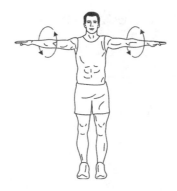

15sec arm circles

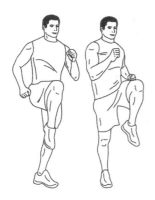

15sec high knees

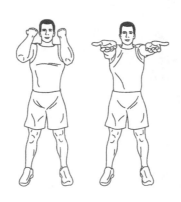

15sec bicep extensions

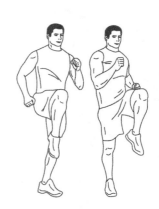

15sec high knees

6 Belly Burner

For those looking for a workout that can help shift those extra few pounds Belly Burner does the trick. Get those knees past your waist each time you do High Knees and make sure you always land on the ball of the foot when you bring your foot down. Go high and fast on the burpees, working your legs to cram in as many reps each time as possible. Recover on the go in-between with elbow plank. Add EC just so you can load your lungs and test your VO2 Max capacity.

Extra Credit: 1 minute rest between sets.

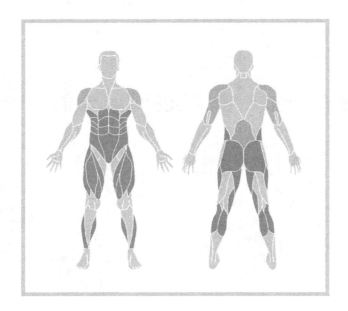

Difficulty

BELLY BURNER

DAREBEE HIIT WORKOUT © darebee.com

Repeat 7 times in total | 2 minutes rest between sets

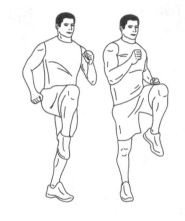

20sec high knees

20sec elbow plank

10sec basic burpees

20sec high knees

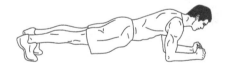

20sec elbow plank

10sec basic burpees

20sec high knees

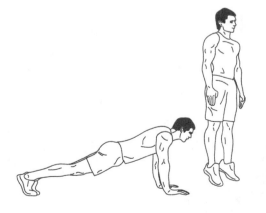

20sec elbow plank

10sec basic burpees

done

7   **Better Tomorrow**

When we do nothing, we only get more of the same. For a better tomorrow, a tomorrow we want to see, we have to apply effort. A better self requires work - through physical work we don't just chisel our bodies, we strengthen our minds, our willpower and resolve. Give it a shot, what do you have to lose? It can only get better.

For best results, go flat out (go as fast as you can) when performing jumping lunges, high knees and jump squats. The workout is designed to go through low-to-high and back to low intervals.

Extra Credit: 1 minute rest between sets.

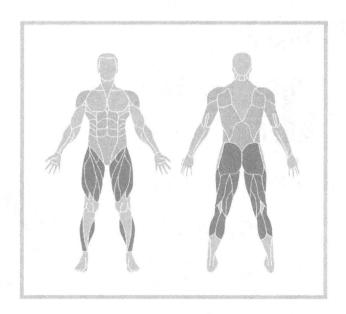

Difficulty

BETTER TOMORROW

DAREBEE **HIIT** WORKOUT © darebee.com

Level I 3 sets **Level II** 5 sets **Level III** 7 sets | 2 minutes rest

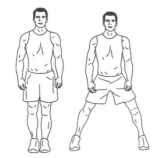

30sec half jacks

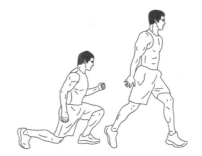

10sec jumping lunges

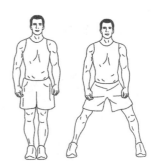

30sec half jacks

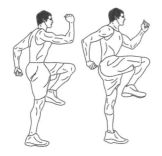

30sec march steps

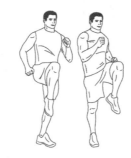

10sec high knees

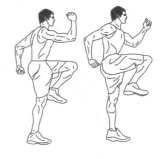

30sec march steps

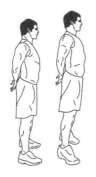

10sec calf raises

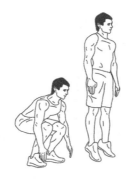

10sec jump squats

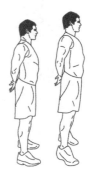

10sec calf raises

8 Blaster

High Intensity Interval Training is not an exercise. It is the furnace where you bake the body you want to have. Sounds like the kind of thing you want to do? Dive into Blaster and be prepared to see some real change, real fast. (You've been warned).

Extra Credit: 30 seconds rest between sets.

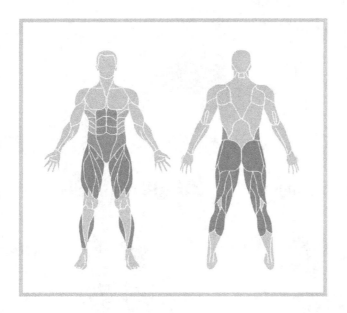

Difficulty

BLASTER

DAREBEE HIIT WORKOUT © darebee.com

Level I 3 sets **Level II** 5 sets **Level III** 7 sets | 2 minutes rest

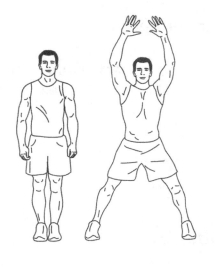

20sec jumping jacks

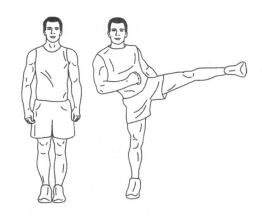

10sec side leg raises

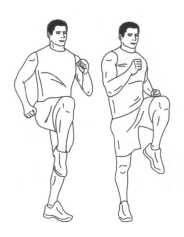

20sec high knees

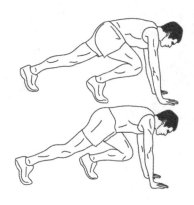

10sec climbers

9 Blueprint

The Blueprint is an aerobic-heavy workout that will raise your body temperature from the first round, push your lungs and test your muscles. As you go from one exercise to the next you alter the load applied to the body's critical muscle groups but you never quite ease it off. The result is a Level 3 workout that will nonetheless push all the right buttons.

Extra Credit: Hit the same number of push-ups and squats every time.

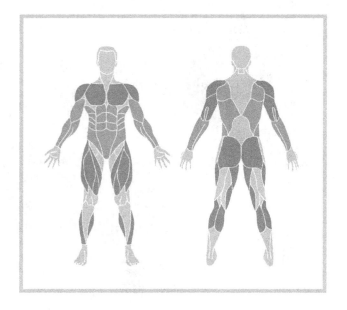

Difficulty

BLUE THE PRINT

DAREBEE HIIT WORKOUT © darebee.com

Level I 3 sets **Level II** 5 sets **Level III** 7 sets | 2 minutes rest

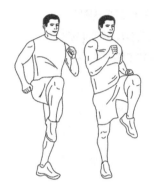
30sec high knees

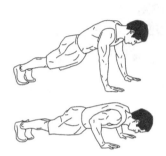
10sec push-ups

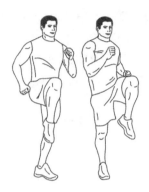
30sec high knees

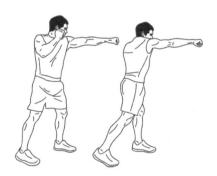
30sec punches

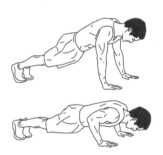
10sec push-ups

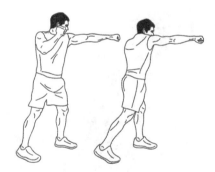
30sec punches

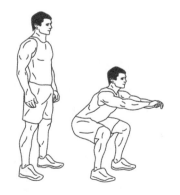
30sec squats

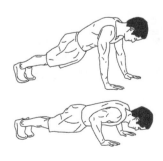
10sec push-ups

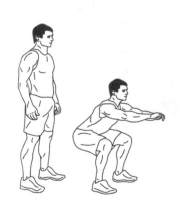
30sec squats

10   **Boiler Room**

Boiler Room lives up to its name by bringing you to the boil in no time at all. It uses every major muscle group in the body piling on the pressure as you go from one exercise to the next. Aim to get in as many reps as possible and try to maintain your performance output steady or increasing as you go from one set to the next.

Extra Credit: Hit the same number of burpees every time.

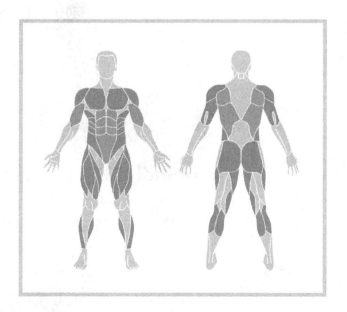

Difficulty

BoilerRoom

DAREBEE HIIT WORKOUT © darebee.com

Level I 3 sets **Level II** 5 sets **Level III** 7 sets **REST** up to 2 minutes rest

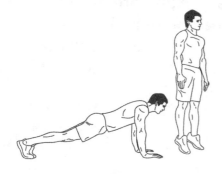

10sec basic burpees

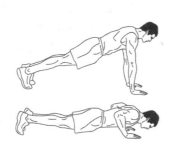

20sec push-ups

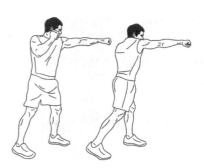

30sec jab + cross

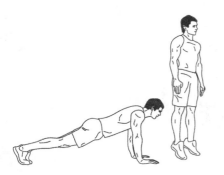

10sec basic burpees

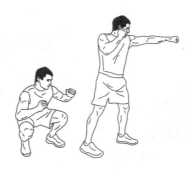

20sec squat + jab

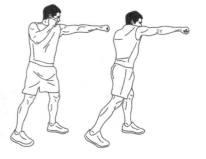

30sec jab + cross

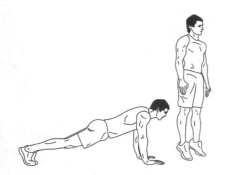

10sec basic burpees

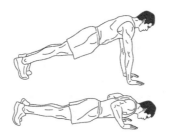

20sec push-ups

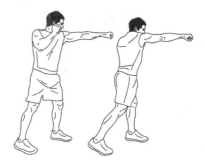

30sec jab + cross

11 Boxer

Boxers have phenomenal limb speed, arm strength and stamina. They can generate tremendous forces on the areas they strike and are easily amongst the most fearsome unarmed fighters anyone can hope to face. The Boxer HIIT workout combines some of the favourite moves of boxing with a high intensity interval training plan that will push your body to its limits.

Extra Credit: 30 seconds rest between sets.

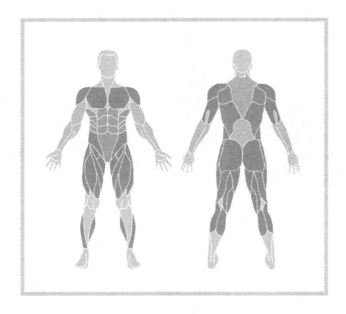

Difficulty

BOXER

DAREBEE HIIT WORKOUT © darebee.com

Level I 3 sets **Level II** 5 sets **Level III** 7 sets | 2 minutes rest

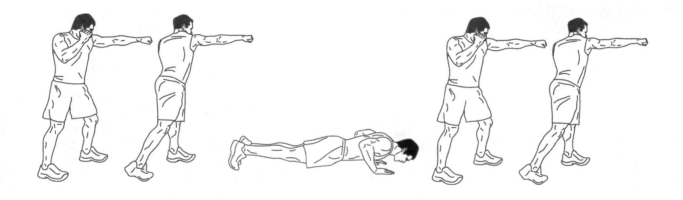

20sec jab + cross   **20sec** push-up + jab + cross

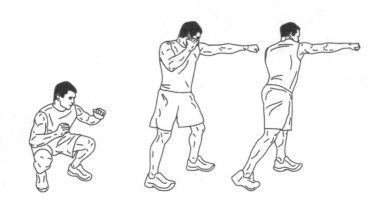

20sec squat + jab + cross

12   **Bulletproof Abs**

Bulletproof Abs is a workout that relentlessly piles up pressure on all major ab wall muscle groups. Perform High Knees by bringing your knee up to waist height each time. Make sure you're on the ball of the foot as you land to absorb the impact from each step. This is a difficulty Level IV workout which means you will definitely feel the burn while doing it.

Extra Credit: 1 minute rest between sets.

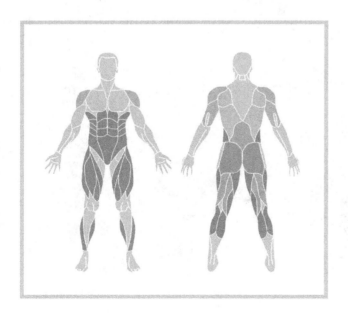

Difficulty

bulletproof abs

HIIT WORKOUT
BY DAREBEE
© darebee.com

Level I 3 sets
Level II 5 sets
Level III 7 sets
2 minutes rest

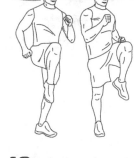

40sec high knees

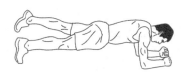

20sec raised leg plank hold (left leg)

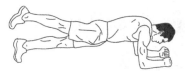

20sec raised leg plank hold (right leg)

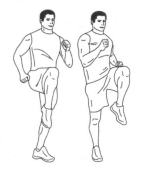

40sec high knees

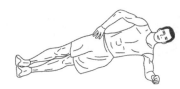

20sec side plank hold (left side)

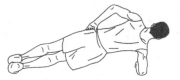

20sec side plank hold (right side)

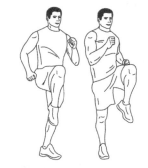

40sec high knees

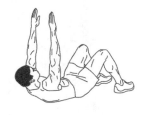

20sec crunch hold

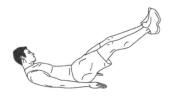

20sec raised leg hold

13 Burn Mode

Jumping Jacks may seem an unlikely exercise to seriously challenge our VO2 Max levels, but performed fast, with perfect form, the heels of the feet never touching down and hands meeting overhead, it becomes key to developing fast, tight, arms/legs coordination and great fascial fitness. Plus there are those core exercises in between that make Burn Mode one to come back to again and again and attempt to conquer at Level III with EC.

Extra Credit: 1 minute rest between sets.

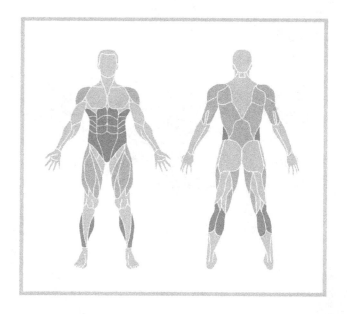

Difficulty

BURN MODE

HIIT WORKOUT
BY DAREBEE
© darebee.com
Level I 3 sets
Level II 5 sets
Level III 7 sets
2 minutes rest

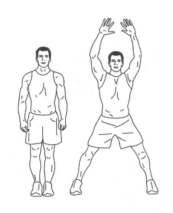

30sec jumping jacks

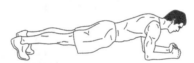

30sec elbow plank

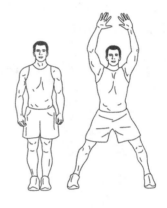

30sec jumping jacks

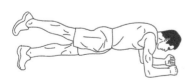

30sec raised leg plank

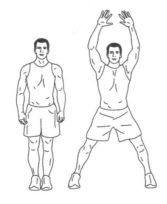

30sec jumping jacks

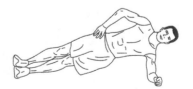

30sec side plank

14 Burn Zone

Burn Zone is a workout designed to get you into the sweat zone from the very first set. Reps count here which means you need to make every second count. Have quick transitions from one exercise to the next. Stay on the balls of your feet during Jumping Jacks and bring your knees to your chest when doing Burpees with Jump Knee Tucks. Stay on the balls of your feet when you land from the Knee Tucks. This is a workout that will test your VO2 Max. Add EC and it becomes a massive challenge.

Extra Credit: 1 minute rest between sets.

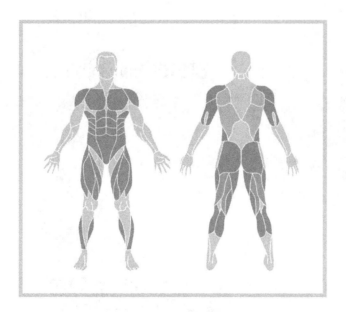

Difficulty

Burn Zone

DAREBEE HIIT WORKOUT © darebee.com

Level I 3 sets **Level II** 5 sets **Level III** 7 sets | 2 minutes rest

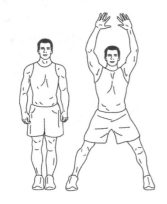

30sec jumping jacks

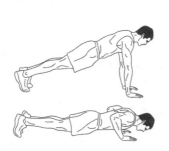

10sec push-ups

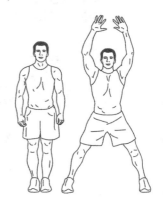

30sec jumping jacks

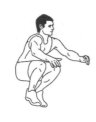
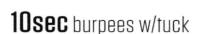

10sec burpees w/tuck

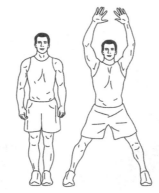

30sec jumping jacks

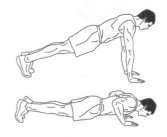

10sec push-ups

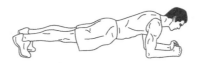

30sec elbow plank

15   Cardio Dive

The abdominal group is made of four separate muscle groups and Cardio Dive is designed to target them all, beginning to increase the load with each set without neglecting the other muscle groups in the body. The result is a seemingly simple workout that gets you sweating quickly and pushes your VO2 Max levels. Make sure you pump your arms during High Knees and you bring your knees to waist height each time.

Extra Credit: 1 minute rest between sets.

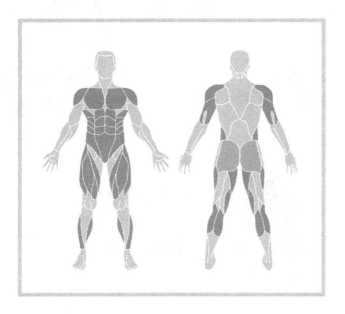

Difficulty

Cardio Dive

DAREBEE **HIIT** WORKOUT © darebee.com

Level I 3 sets **Level II** 5 sets **Level III** 7 sets

2 minutes rest between sets

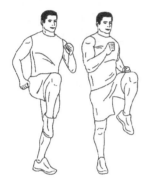

20sec high knees

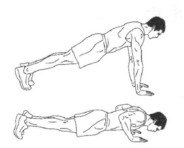

20sec push-ups

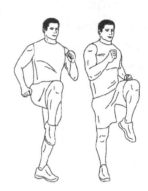

20sec high knees

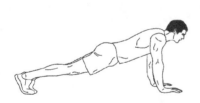

20sec plank

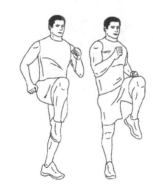

20sec high knees

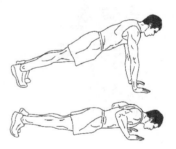

20sec push-ups

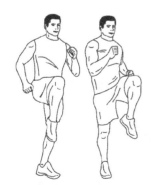

20sec high knees

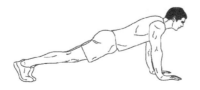

20sec plank

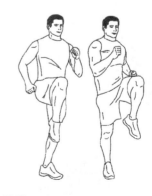

20sec high knees

16 Cardio Mixer

Before our roaming plane of existence was bounded by the walls of our office space, life was punctuated by short, sharp bursts of activity as we hunted for food and fought for territory. We no longer have to do any of that but a short, sharp burst of intense activity still makes us feel alive.

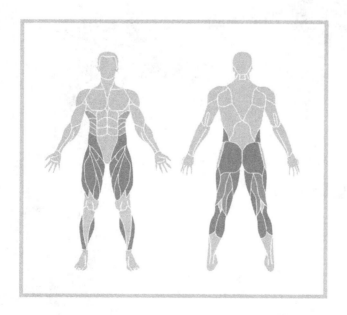

Difficulty

Cardio Mixer

DAREBEE HIIT WORKOUT © darebee.com

Level I 3 sets **Level II** 5 sets **Level III** 7 sets | 2 minutes rest

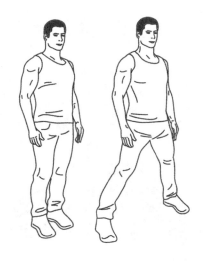

20sec half jacks

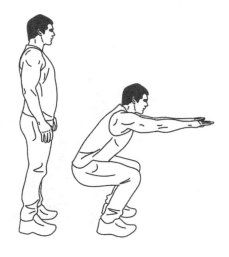

20sec squats

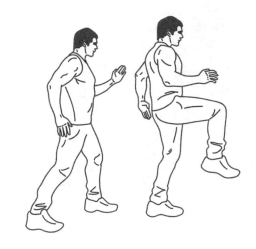

20sec step back + knee ups

Cardio Prime

You barely need any space for this high intensity, interval training workout. You could almost perform it standing in a barrel which means you now have no real excuses for not trying this at least once.

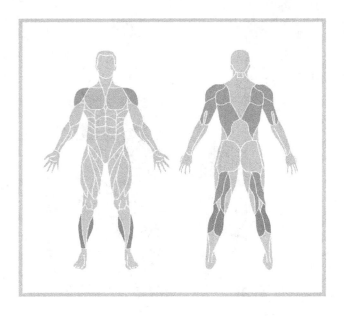

Difficulty

Cardio Prime

DAREBEE HIIT WORKOUT © darebee.com

Level I 3 sets **Level II** 5 sets **Level III** 7 sets | 2 minutes rest

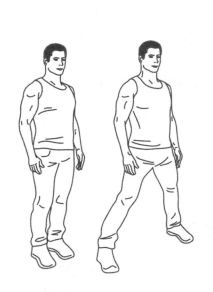 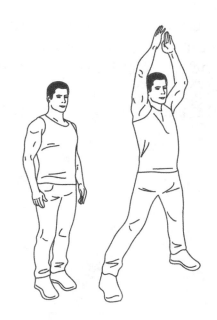

10sec half jacks

10sec jumping jacks

10sec half jacks

10sec jumping jacks

10sec half jacks

10sec jumping jacks

done

18 Cardio Pro

Cardio Pro is a High Intensity Interval Training Program designed to help your body burn high and your muscles work hard. The exercise transition allows for some recovery on the fly while the load to the muscle groups being worked is applied with some consistency throughout each set and with higher intensity at specific moments in the set. Add EC to challenge yourself and try to extend the reach of your physical prowess.

Extra Credit: Hit the same number of basic burpees every time.

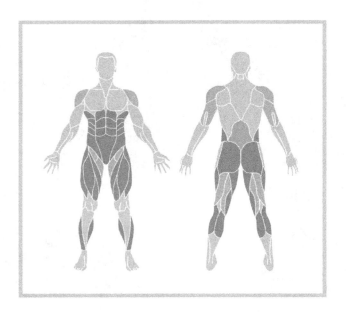

Difficulty

Cardio Pro

DAREBEE `HIIT` WORKOUT © darebee.com

Level I 3 sets **Level II** 5 sets **Level III** 7 sets

2 minutes rest rest between sets

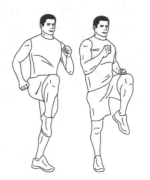

30sec high knees

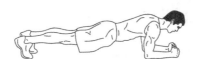

30sec elbow plank

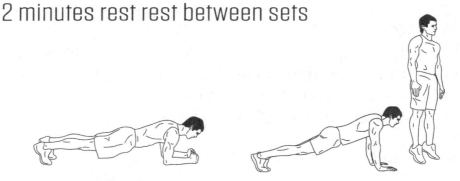

10sec basic burpees

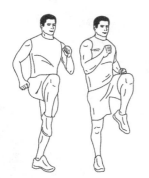

30sec high knees

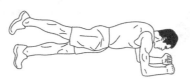

30sec raised leg plank

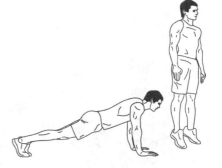

10sec basic burpees

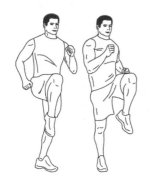

30sec high knees

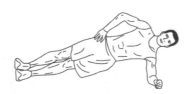

30sec side elbow plank

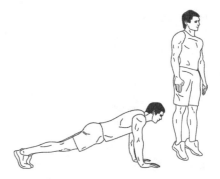

10sec basic burpees

19   Carpe Diem

If seizing the day is your thing then Carpe Diem should be your workout. This is a high-speed, high-intensity, Level IV workout that will put you in the sweatzone from the very first set and keep you there for every set after that. Get your knees to waist height during High Knees and don't forget to pump your arms. Everything is time-based which means that reps really matter. Try to get as many as you can in each exercise and maintain or improve the level in each set. Add EC (you will really know the burn then).

Extra Credit: 1 minute rest between sets.

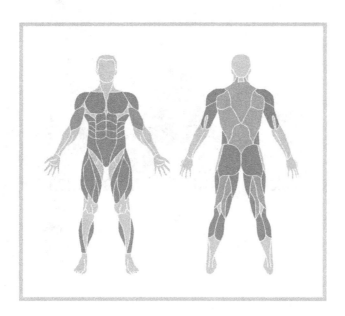

Difficulty

CARPE DIEM

DAREBEE HIIT WORKOUT © darebee.com

Level I 3 sets **Level II** 5 sets **Level III** 7 sets | 2 minutes rest

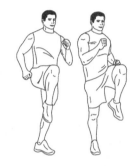

20sec high knees

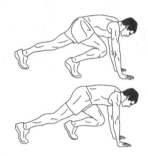

20sec climbers

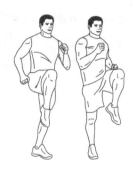

20sec high knees

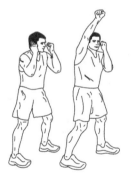

20sec overhead punches

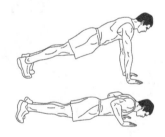

20sec push-ups

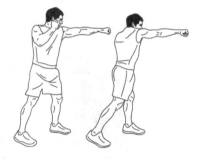

20sec punches

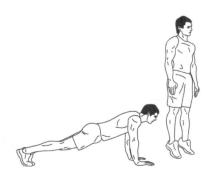

20sec basic burpees

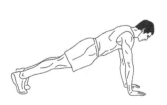

20sec plank hold

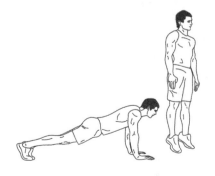

20sec basic burpees

20 The Catch

The Catch is not difficult. In fact as a difficulty Level II workout it will just keep you ticking over on the days when you just cannot get sufficient drive to explore the limits of what you can do. But on those days this is exactly what you need in order to maintain the momentum of your fitness journey. You know the drill. Be light on your feet when you're doing Jumping Ts and maintain a straight body during the plank.

Extra Credit: 1 minute rest between sets.

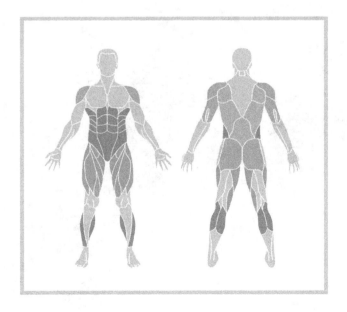

Difficulty

THE CATCH

DAREBEE **HIIT** WORKOUT © darebee.com

Level I 3 sets **Level II** 5 sets **Level III** 7 sets | 2 minutes rest

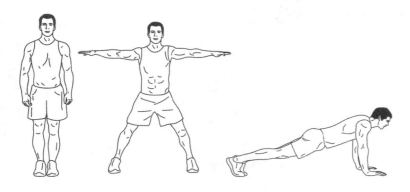

30sec jumping Ts   **30sec** plank

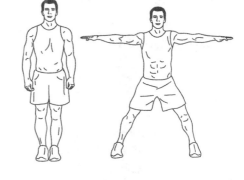

30sec jumping Ts

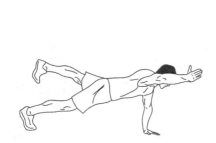

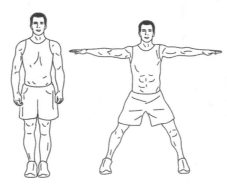

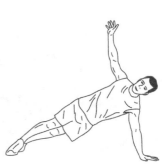

30sec alt arm/leg plank   **30sec** jumping Ts   **30sec** one-arm side plank

21   Chisel Express

When we listen to our body we know when there are days when all we need is a fast, energizing workout that will not take us to the very brink of our resources but will still leave us feeling like we've worked out. Chisel is just such a workout. It uses just three basic bodyweight exercises in a combination that is challenging enough to help us shape our body and see results. Being a Level II workout however this is the one you do when you are "building up" to greater things or "powering down" and maintaining your edge on days when you're not in your top form.

Extra Credit: 1 minute rest between sets.

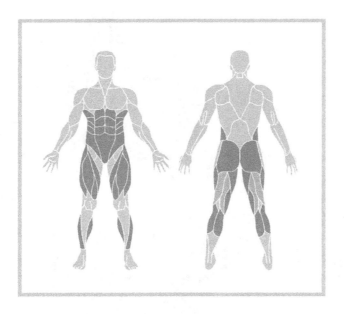

Difficulty

CHISEL

EXPRESS

DAREBEE **HIIT** WORKOUT © darebee.com

Level I 3 sets **Level II** 5 sets **Level III** 7 sets | 2 minutes rest rest

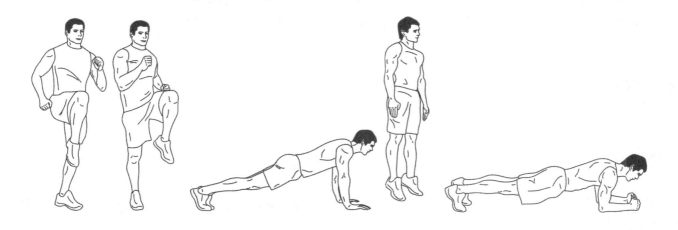

20sec high knees

10sec basic burpees

20sec high knees

10sec basic burpees

20sec high knees

10sec basic burpees

30sec elbow plank

done

22 Chopper

If someone urges you to get to the chopper you know it ain't going to be easy. For a start just calling it "chopper" means you're in a tight spot with time running out and the hordes bearing down upon you. Plus you're probably out of ammo and have nowhere to hide either. Good thing the Get To The Chopper workout is here to help you get fit enough to make it before they get you. EC is a must here. You never know when you just may need to extra boost.

Extra Credit: 1 minute rest between sets.

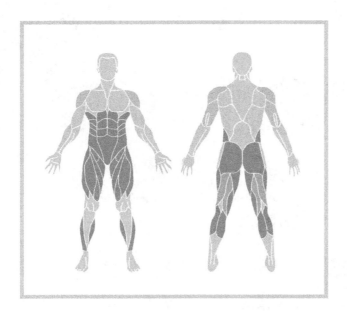

Difficulty

get to the chopper

DAREBEE HIIT WORKOUT © darebee.com

Level I 3 sets **Level II** 5 sets **Level III** 7 sets | 2 minutes rest

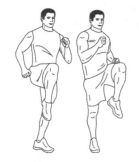

20sec high knees

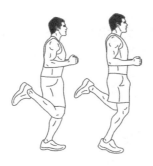

20sec butt kicks

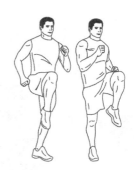

20sec high knees

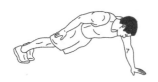

20sec one-arm plank

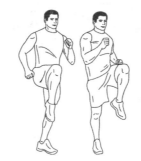

20sec high knees

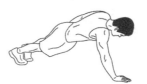

20sec one-arm plank

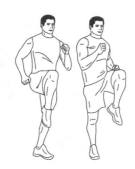

20sec high knees

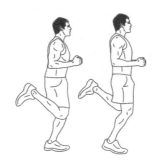

20sec butt kicks

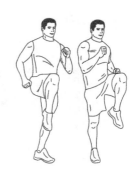

20sec high knees

23 Coda

Take your cardio to the next level with the CODA workout. It has the best of everything and it has the worst of everything - catch your breath and dare it again! Who Dares, Wins.

Extra Credit: Keep the plank throughout the second row.

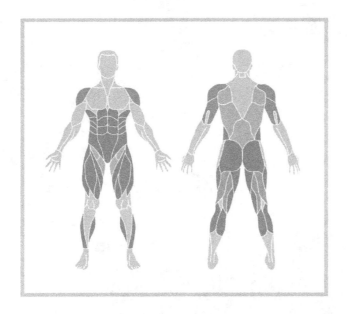

Difficulty

CODA

DAREBEE `HIIT` WORKOUT © darebee.com

Level I 3 sets **Level II** 5 sets **Level III** 7 sets | 2 minutes rest

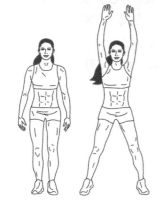

20sec jumping jacks

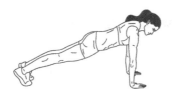

20sec plank hold

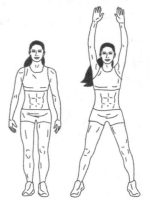

20sec jumping jacks

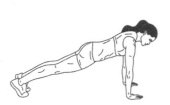

20sec plank hold

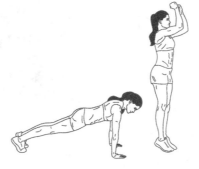

20sec basic burpees

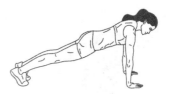

20sec plank hold

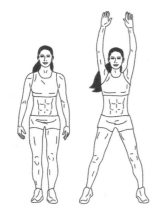

20sec jumping jacks

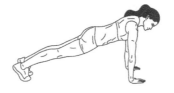

20sec plank hold

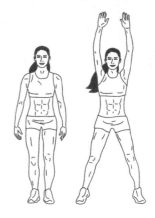

20sec jumping jacks

24   **Combat Burpee**

Halloween is rock candy night which means "zero guilt" for you provided you do the Combat Burpee workout. A difficulty Level IV workout, it is designed to help you get that extra burn which probably makes it a great primer to that night out when you know you won't be able to turn down dessert.

Extra Credit: 1 minute rest between sets.

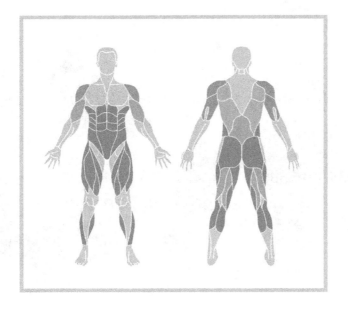

Difficulty

combat burpee

DAREBEE HIIT WORKOUT © darebee.com

Level I 3 sets • **Level II** 5 sets **Level III** 7 sets | 2 minutes rest

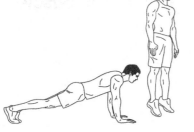

20sec basic burpees

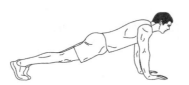

10sec plank hold

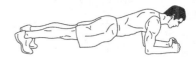

30sec elbow plank hold

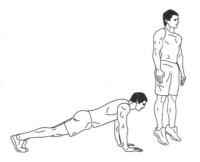

20sec basic burpees

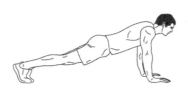

10sec plank hold

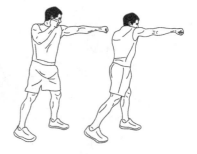

30sec punches

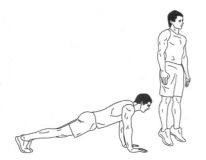

20sec basic burpees

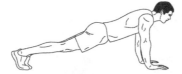

10sec plank hold

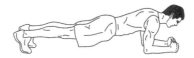

30sec elbow plank hold

25   Confessor

Confessors require agility, speed and razor-sharp reflexes. Mere muscle bulk will not do here. You need tendon strength and muscle density. A body that is balanced and capable. You need to be able to 'dance' through your routine rather than power through it. This workout works the parts of the body that will help you do just that. It is intended to give you control and it allows you to become more powerful by linking up different muscle systems.

Extra Credit: 30 seconds rest between sets.

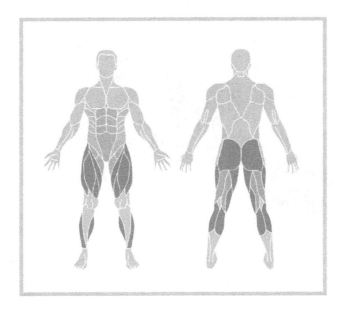

Difficulty

CONFESSOR

DAREBEE HIIT WORKOUT © darebee.com
Level I 3 sets **Level II** 5 sets **Level III** 7 sets | 2 minutes rest

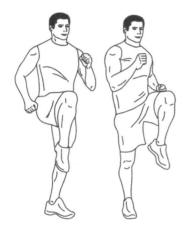

20sec high knees

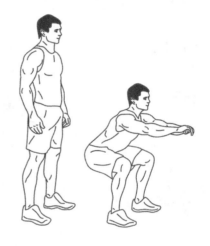

10sec squats

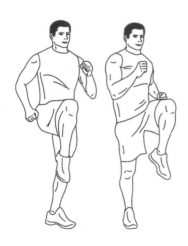

20sec high knees

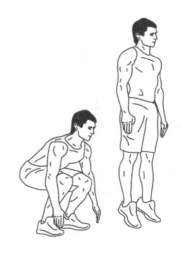

10sec jump squats

26 Core Burn

Core Burn demands perfect form when performing High Knees, which means your knees need to come to waist height each time and you only ever land on the ball of the foot. You pump your arms in synch to your legs. The rest of the exercises are not easy either but then again you're here to make your core and abs feel they've worked out. This will do it.

Extra Credit: 1 minute rest between sets.

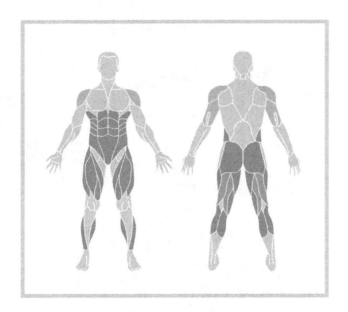

Difficulty

Core Burn

DAREBEE HIIT WORKOUT © darebee.com
Level I 3 sets Level II 5 sets Level III 7 sets
2 minutes rest between sets

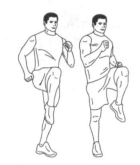

20sec high knees

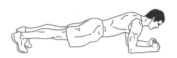

20sec elbow plank

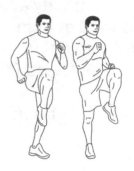

20sec high knees

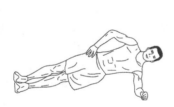

20sec side plank (left)

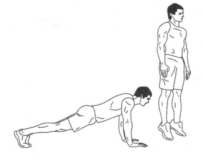

20sec basic burpees

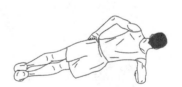

20sec side plank (right)

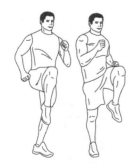

20sec high knees

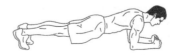

20sec elbow plank

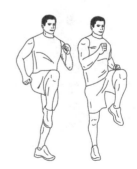

20sec high knees

27 Core Sculpt

Core Sculpt uses High Knees and some basic core training exercises to raise your body temperature, challenge tendon strength and VO2 Max performance and work the main abdominal groups. The floor exercises provide a handy active recovery stage which means High Knees are performed at high intensity with lots of pumping of the arms and with the knees coming up to waist height, each time. Remember to land on the ball of your foot. Add EC, com'on. Add it!

Extra Credit: 1 minute rest between sets.

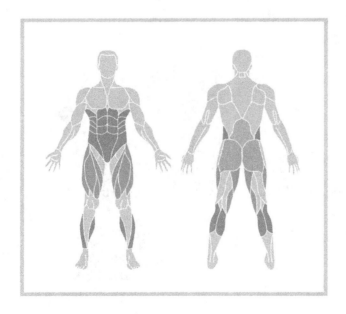

Difficulty

core sculpt

DAREBEE **HIIT** WORKOUT © darebee.com

Level I 3 sets **Level II** 5 sets **Level III** 7 sets

2 minutes rest between sets

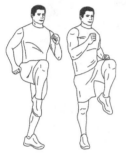

20sec high knees

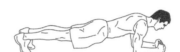

20sec elbow plank

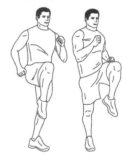

20sec high knees

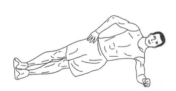

20sec side plank (left)

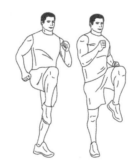

20sec high knees

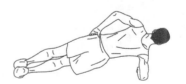

20sec side plank (right)

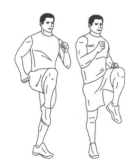

20sec high knees

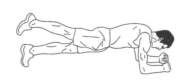

20sec raised leg elbow plank

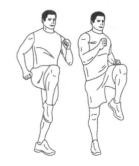

20sec high knees

28   **Crossfire**

The real meaning of this workout becomes evident only after you've blasted through it a few times. This is a High Intensity Interval Training that'll leave you feeling like you can take on the world, once you've caught your breath. If you ever find yourself in a crossfire.

Extra Credit: 30 seconds rest between sets.

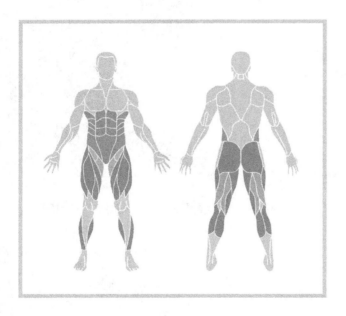

Difficulty

CROSSFIRE

DAREBEE HIIT WORKOUT © darebee.com

Level I 3 sets **Level II** 5 sets **Level III** 7 sets | 2 minutes rest

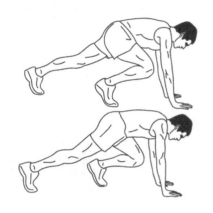

20sec climbers

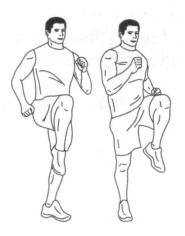

10sec high knees

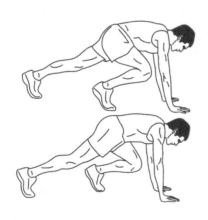

10sec climbers

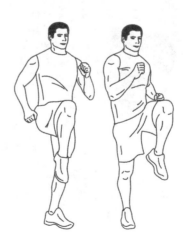

20sec high knees

29   Cursor

If what you are looking for is a workout that transforms your entire body into an instrument to be used by you then you need go no further than Cursor. Utilizing a combination of concentric and eccentric muscle movements, performed at speed, and using all of the body's major muscle groups Cursor becomes the workout that tests your capability and keeps on testing it until you've mastered it, which means Level III, with EC and finishing with some spare energy in the tank.

Extra Credit: Hit the same number of jumping lunges each time.

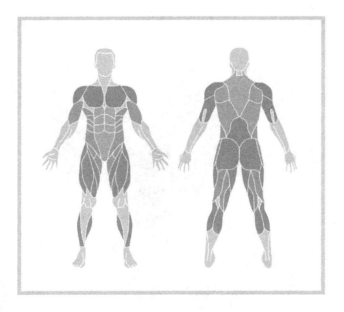

Difficulty

cursor

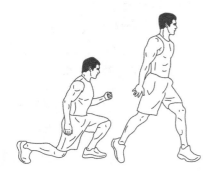

10sec jumping lunges

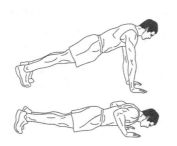

10sec push-ups

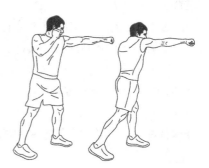

40sec punches

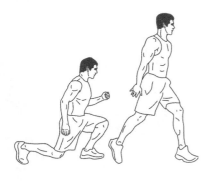

10sec jumping lunges

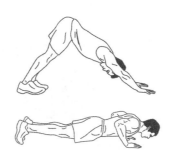

10sec judo push-ups

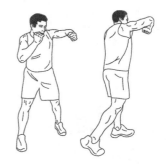

40sec hooks

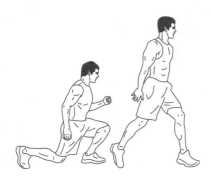

10sec jumping lunges

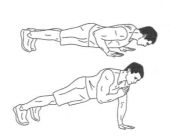

10sec push-up + shoulder tap

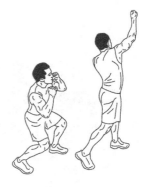

40sec uppercuts

30 Double Helix

Double Helix is a game of two halves. You work the lower body, transferring the load to the upper body and then you take it back to the lower body again and in all this time your core and abs are working hard. This is a full body HIIT workout that will get you in the sweat zone from the very first set. Go for the maximum rep count in each exercise use EC as a measure of your fitness level.

Extra Credit: Hit the same number of push-ups each time.

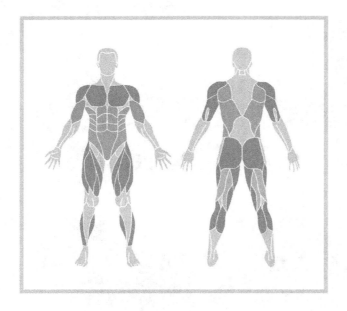

Difficulty

DOUBLE HELIX

DAREBEE `HIIT` WORKOUT © darebee.com

LEVEL I 3 sets **LEVEL II** 5 sets **LEVEL III** 7 sets **REST** up to 2 minutes

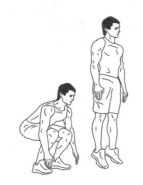
10sec jump squats

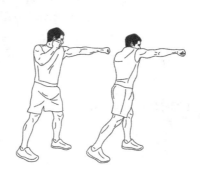
40sec punches

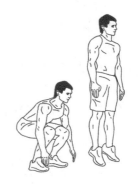
10sec jump squats

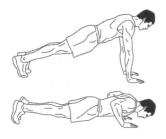
10sec push-ups

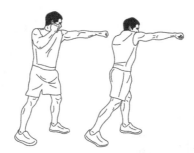
40sec punches

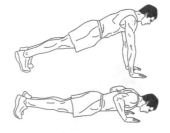
10sec push-ups

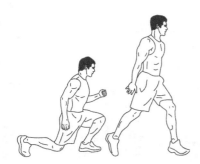
10sec jumping lunges

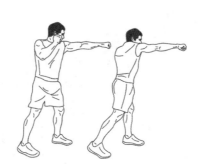
40sec punches

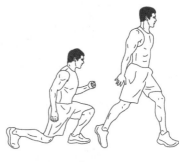
10sec jumping lunges

31 **Drifter**

The Drifter is only a difficulty Level II workout. That makes it light and fast, relying on constant motion to raise your body temperature and bring you to the sweatzone. Keep on the balls of your feet when you do Jumping Jacks and really work your arms and legs fast. Try to get a high rep count on every exercise and then maintain it on each set.

Extra Credit: 1 minute rest between sets.

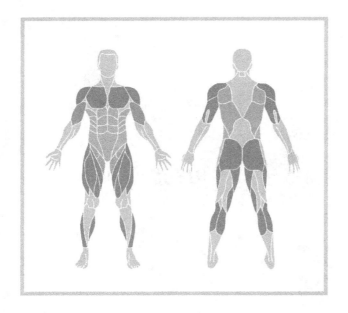

Difficulty

THE DRIFTER

DAREBEE `HIIT` WORKOUT © darebee.com

Level I 3 sets **Level II** 5 sets **Level III** 7 sets | 2 minutes rest

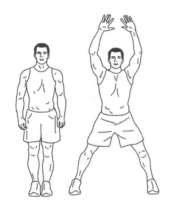

20sec jumping jacks

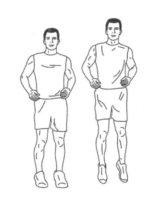

20sec hops on the spot

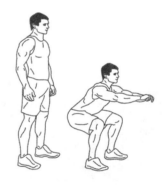

20sec squats

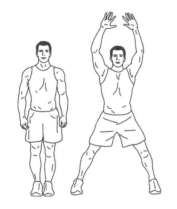

20sec jumping jacks

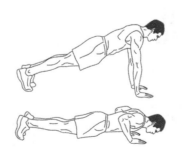

20sec push-ups

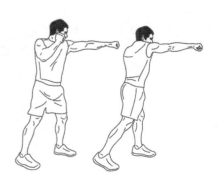

20sec punches

32   Expedited Delivery

Expedited delivery is zippy and even the floor exercises are designed to put a load on muscles ans tendons that are used in the rest of the workout. That makes it a challenge to get through without a groan 9or two) which means it will work to bring up your body temperature and put you in the sweatzone, fast.

Extra Credit: 1 minute rest between sets.

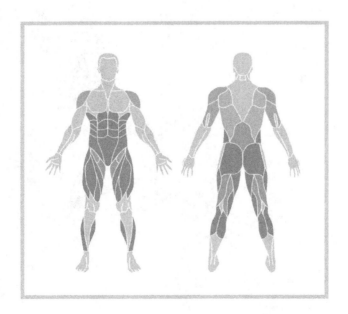

Difficulty

EXPEDITED DELIVERY

DAREBEE `HIIT` WORKOUT © darebee.com

Level I 3 sets **Level II** 5 sets **Level III** 7 sets | 2 minutes rest

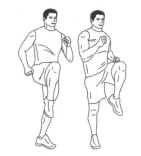

20sec high knees

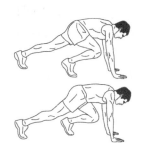

20sec climbers

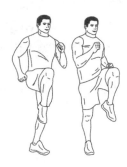

20sec high knees

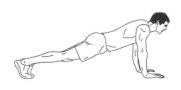

20sec plank hold

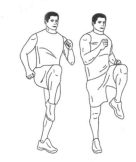

20sec high knees

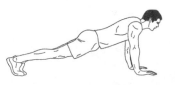

20sec plank hold

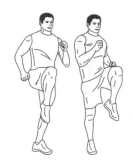

20sec high knees

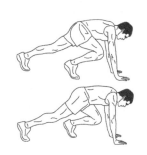

20sec climbers

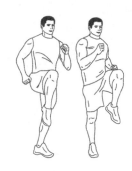

20sec high knees

33   Fab Abs

The abs and core are the junction at which lower body strength is translated into upper body power. But for that to happen you need strong abs and a strong core. Fab Abs works all of that in a dynamic and static fashion. The cross-mix delivers a potent abs workout that demands you raise your knees to waist height during High Knees and keep your body as absolutely straight as you possibly can during plank. Add EC when you need the extra challenge that will make your abs and core burn.

Extra Credit: 1 minute rest between sets.

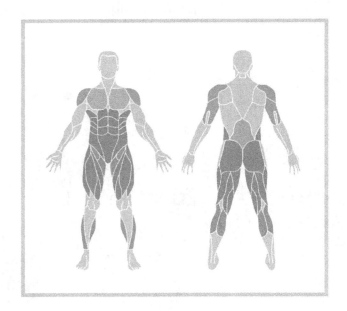

Difficulty

FAB ABS

DAREBEE HIIT WORKOUT © darebee.com

Level I 3 sets **Level II** 5 sets **Level III** 7 sets | 2 minutes rest

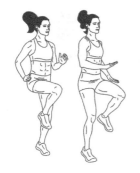
20sec high knees

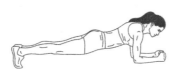
20sec elbow plank hold

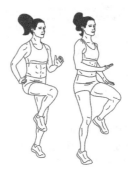
20sec high knees

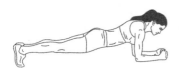
20sec elbow plank hold

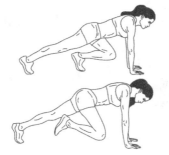
20sec climbers

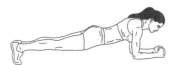
20sec elbow plank hold

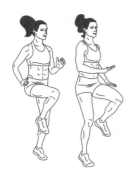
20sec high knees

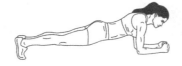
20sec elbow plank hold

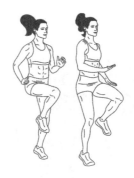
20sec high knees

Fast & Dangerous

A fast burst of activity is all it takes to get your body moving, your heart pumping and your brain racing. You actually need all of this to get through a productive day and you can gain a real boost by investing just 60 seconds of your time (of course you can repeat again and again).

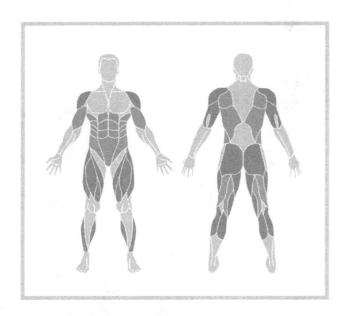

Difficulty

Fast & Dangerous

DAREBEE HIIT WORKOUT © darebee.com

Level I 3 sets **Level II** 5 sets **Level III** 7 sets | 2 minutes rest

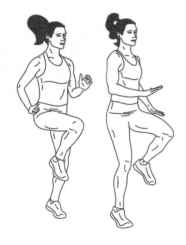

15sec high knees

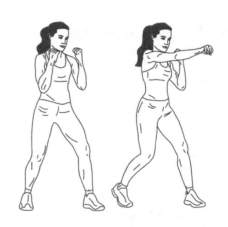

15sec punches

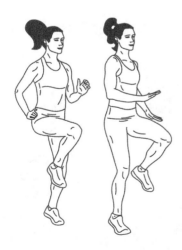

15sec high knees

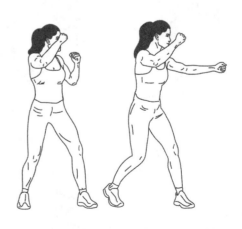

15sec backfists

35 Fire Punch

The Fire Punch workout, as expected, puts some fire back into your punches. Punches are not made in the biceps. or even the shoulders. It takes strong legs and a good core to drive them home. The Fire Punch workout delivers on all those fronts. Add EC and you're also testing your aerobic capacity.

Extra Credit: 1 minute rest between sets.

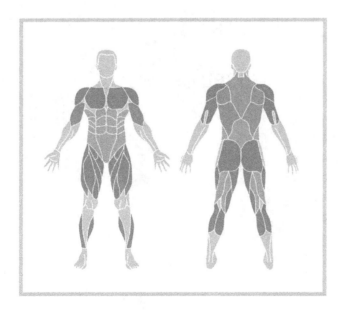

Difficulty

FIRE PUNCH

DAREBEE HIIT WORKOUT © darebee.com

Level I 3 sets **Level II** 5 sets **Level III** 7 sets | 2 minutes rest

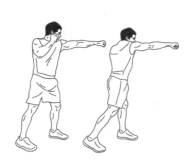

20sec punches

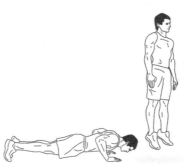

20sec burpees

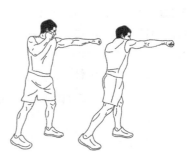

20sec punches

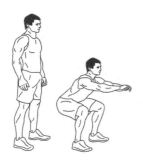

20sec squats

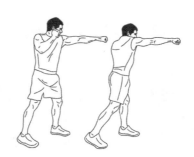

20sec punches

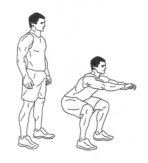

20sec squats

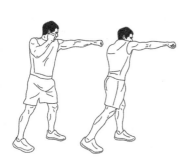

20sec punches

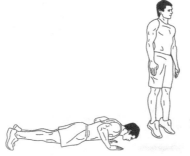

20sec burpees

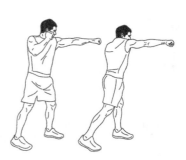

20sec punches

36 Flamethrower

How tough are you? Really? The Flamethrower workout is one way to find out. Beyond the need to really pack in the reps count in every 15-second segment there is the requirement to really keep those knees waist-high for 30 seconds at a time. This is a high burn workout that gets you into the sweat zone very, very quickly and then simply does not let up. Like any Level four difficulty, workout it requires you to stay focused and on form and try to maintain your rep count the same throughout.

Extra Credit: Hit the same number of push-ups every time.

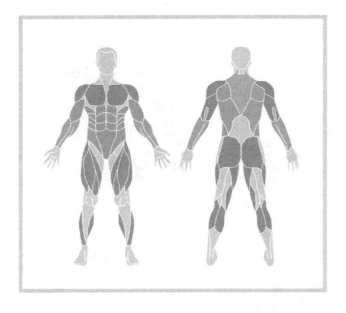

Difficulty

FLAMETHROWER

DAREBEE `HIIT` WORKOUT © darebee.com

Level I 3 sets **Level II** 5 sets **Level III** 7 sets **REST** up to 2 minutes rest

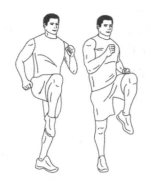
30sec high knees

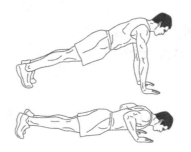
15sec push-ups

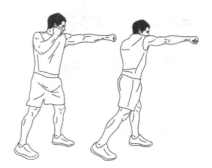
15sec jab + cross

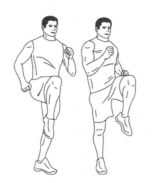
30sec high knees

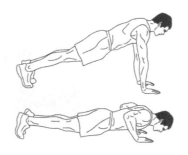
15sec push-ups

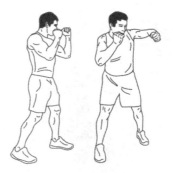
15sec hooks

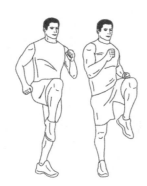
30sec high knees

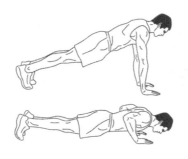
15sec push-ups

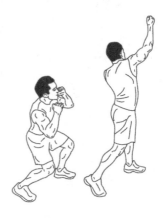
15sec uppercuts

37 Flyby

Keep on the balls of your feet when doing Jumping Jacks and this workout begins to get way harder than it has any right to be. You're on a time limit on each exercise so the number of reps really counts, try to get as many in each exercise segment as possible and keep the number consistent throughout.

Extra Credit: Keep the plank changing from plank to raised leg plank.

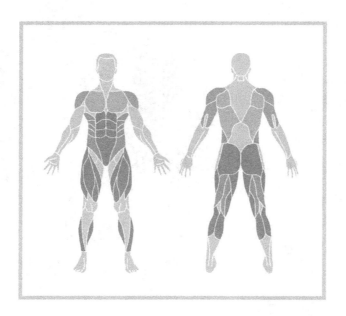

Difficulty

FLYBY

DAREBEE `HIIT` WORKOUT © darebee.com

Level I 3 sets **Level II** 5 sets **Level III** 7 sets | 2 minutes rest

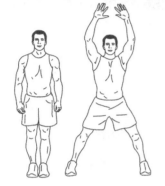

20sec jumping jacks

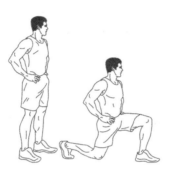

20sec lunges

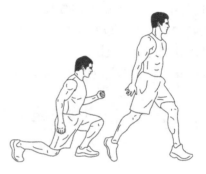

20sec jumping lunges

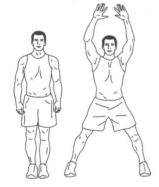

20sec jumping jacks

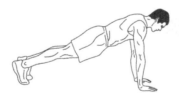

20sec plank

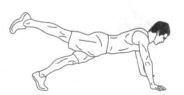

20sec raised leg plank

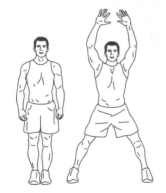

20sec jumping jacks

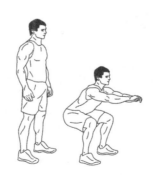

20sec squats

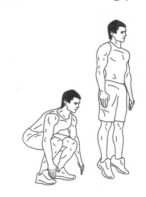

20sec jump squats

38 Free Fall

Free Fall is an aerobic-heavy HIIT workout that works hard to bring fascial fitness levels up, increase upper/lower body synchronization and deliver a strong core. It gets you into the sweat zone from the first three and a half minutes and then it keeps you there. Test your performance by counting what you do on each exercise in your first two sets and then see if you can maintain it throughout the number of sets you do. Extra Credit given if you manage this on burpees.

Extra Credit: hit the same number of basic burpees every time.

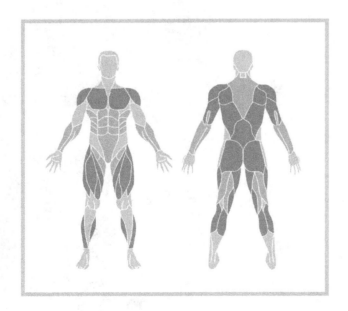

Difficulty

FREE FALL

DAREBEE **HIIT** WORKOUT

© **darebee.com**

Level I 3 sets
Level II 5 sets
Level III 7 sets
2 minutes rest between sets

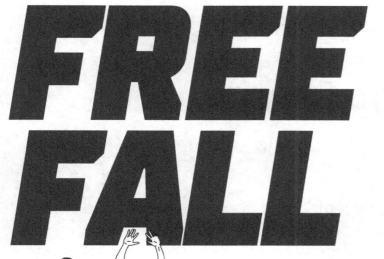

30sec jumping jacks   **30sec** basic burpees   **30sec** raised arm circles

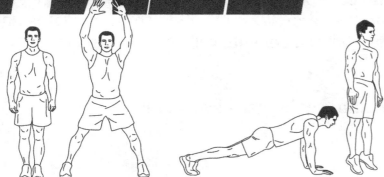
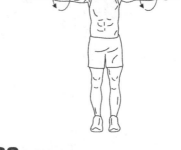

30sec jumping jacks   **30sec** basic burpees   **30sec** raised arm circles

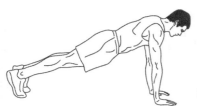
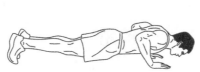
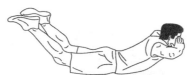

20sec push-up into back extension   +   **10sec** back extension hold

39 Game Changer

Through a series of successive eccentric and concentric exercises coupled with upper body and core-challenging work, the Game Changer workout succeeds in loading the cardiovascular and aerobic systems and establishing a training routine whose benefits will not take long to make themselves felt.

Extra Credit: Hit the same number of burpees every time.

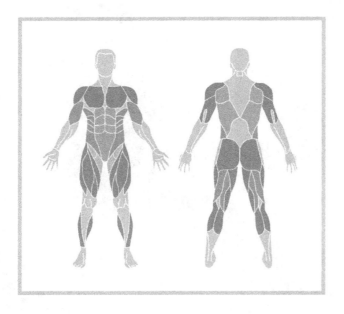

Difficulty

Game Changer

DAREBEE `HIIT` WORKOUT © darebee.com

Level I 3 sets **Level II** 5 sets **Level III** 7 sets | 2 minutes rest

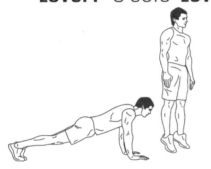

15sec basic burpees

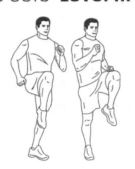

30sec high knees

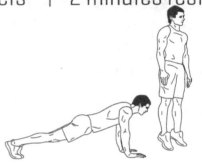

15sec basic burpees

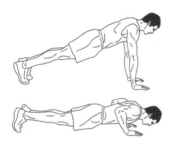

15sec push-ups

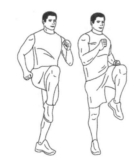

30sec high knees

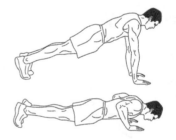

15sec push-ups

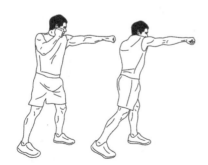

15sec punches

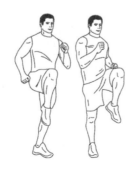

30sec high knees

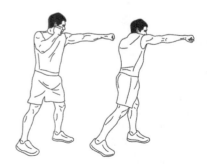

15sec punches

40 Genesis

It's always hard in the beginning but if you stick with it, in the end it's all worth it. The Genesis workout is pure fire, it will break you to remake you. Bear with it, give it your all, persevere and, once you conquer it, nothing will ever feel like too much to overcome. This is how toughness is nurtured and how iron will is forged. Keep moving, as fast as you can until the time is done, catch your breath and do it again. Bring your knees up as high as you can, as far in as you can and don't forget to breathe!

Extra Credit: 1 minute rest between sets.

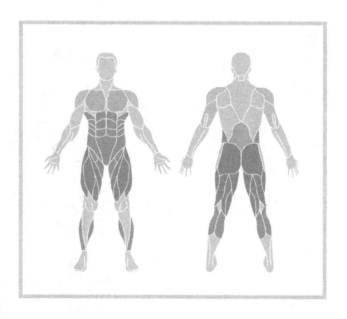

Difficulty

GENESIS

DAREBEE `HIIT` WORKOUT © darebee.com

Level I 3 sets **Level II** 5 sets **Level III** 7 sets | 2 minutes rest

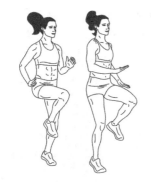

20sec high knees

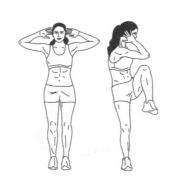

20sec knee-to-elbows

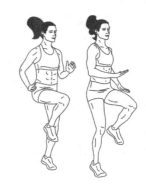

20sec high knees

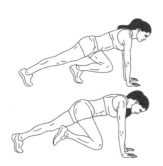

20sec climbers

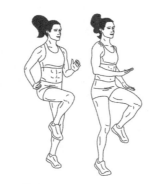

20sec high knees

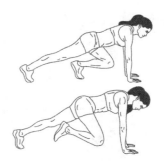

20sec climbers

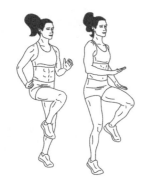

20sec high knees

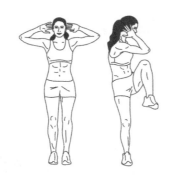

20sec knee-to-elbows

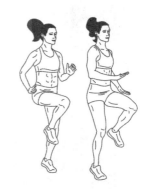

20sec high knees

Get It Done

This workout is perfect for when you just need to - Get It Done. It will challenge your lungs and work your core without overtaxing your system delivering just the right amount of burn, at the right time. It's fairly easy to follow, there are no complex moves, but it will work your entire body nonetheless. Keep your arm up throughout the second row and keep your elbows pointing forward during bicep extensions - don't drop your arms down, for maximum results.

Extra Credit: 1 minute rest between sets.

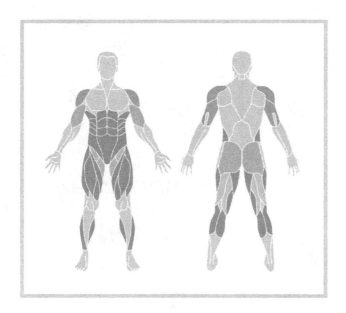

Difficulty

Get It Done

DAREBEE `HIIT` WORKOUT © darebee.com

Level I 3 sets **Level II** 5 sets **Level III** 7 sets

2 minutes rest between sets

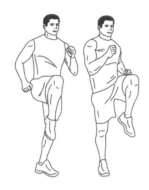
20sec high knees

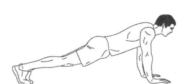
20sec plank hold

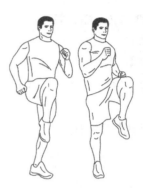
20sec high knees

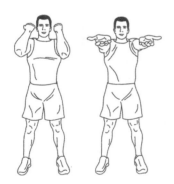
20sec bicep extensions

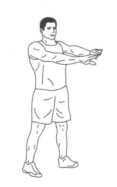
20sec raised arm hold

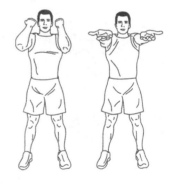
20sec bicep extensions

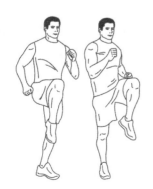
20sec high knees

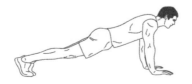
20sec plank hold

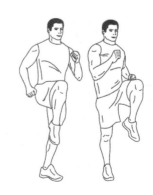
20sec high knees

42 Grasshopper

Use your body to fight gravity and develop the kind of elastic, explosive, lean muscle that makes you feel like you can do anything. Grasshopper is just such a workout. It helps you develop fascial strength and it still takes you to the point where your VO2 Max is challenged. Add EC and you have a real winner on your hands.

Extra Credit: 1 minute rest between sets.

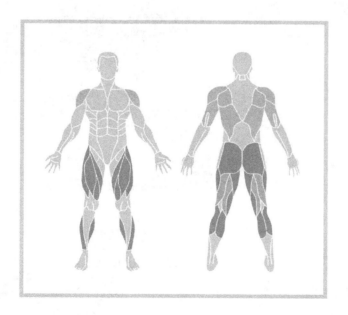

Difficulty

GRASSHOPPER

DAREBEE HIIT WORKOUT © darebee.com

Level I 3 sets **Level II** 5 sets **Level III** 7 sets | 2 minutes rest

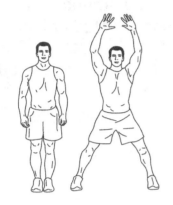
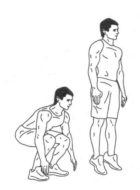

60sec jumping jacks
one jump squat
every 15 seconds

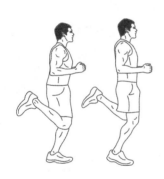
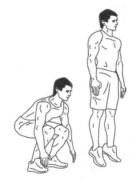

60sec butt kicks
one jump squat
every 15 seconds

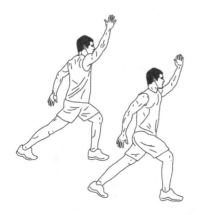
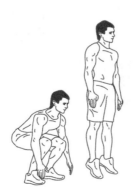

60sec split jacks
one jump squat
every 15 seconds

43 Grind

If you're going to hone your body to a fine edge you need an exceptional grind. The Grind is a workout that helps you develop lower body strength and total body coordination. The difficulty level may not be very high but that doesn't mean that the intensity is not there. Pick your knees up to waist height each time you step, work your arms in coordinated unison and feel the difference it all makes to the way your body functions. Great for those just starting out but also a perfect tuner-upper for those who need a workout on days when they don't always feel like going flat-out.

Extra Credit: 1 minute rest between sets.

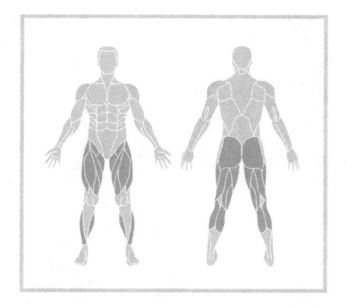

Difficulty

THE GRIND

DAREBEE HIIT WORKOUT © darebee.com

Level I 3 sets **Level II** 5 sets **Level III** 7 sets | 2 minutes rest

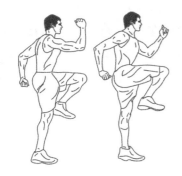

30sec march steps

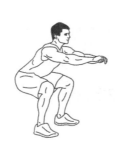

10sec squat hold

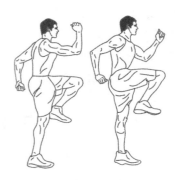

30sec march steps

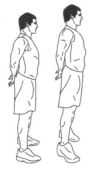

10sec calf raises

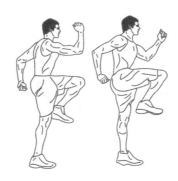

30sec march steps

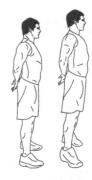

10sec calf raises

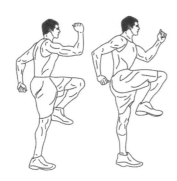

30sec march steps

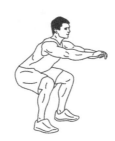

10sec squat hold

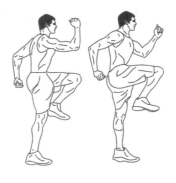

30sec march steps

44   **Hear Me Roar**

Hear Me Roar is the kind of workout that pushes you into the sweat zone within the first three minutes of exercise (which is the first set). It engages core, upper body and lower body, equally - engaging all the major muscle groups it places quite a load on aerobic performance (VO2 Max). Performed at Level III with EC this is workout designed to push the boundaries of physical performance.

Extra Credit: 1 push-ups every 20 seconds

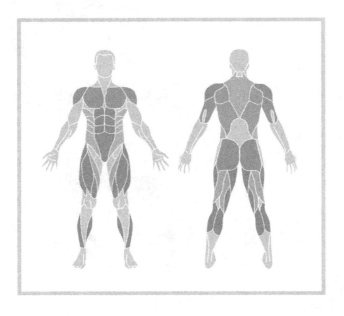

Difficulty

Hear Me Roar

DAREBEE HIIT WORKOUT © darebee.com

Level I 3 rounds   Level II 5 rounds   Level III 7 rounds   2 min rest between rounds

Extra Credit   1 push-up every 20 seconds

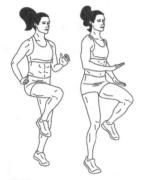
20sec high knees

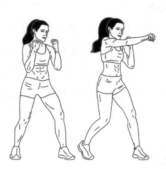
20sec punches

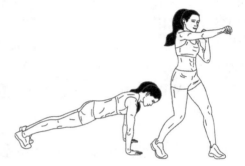
20sec plank + jab + cross

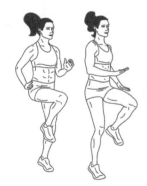
20sec high knees

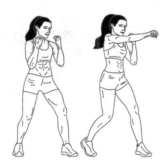
20sec punches

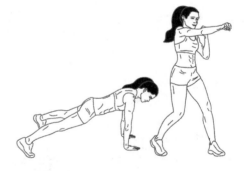
20sec plank jack + jab + cross

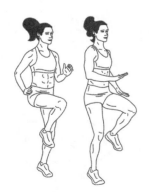
20sec high knees

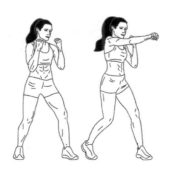
20sec punches

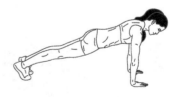
finish 20sec plank

45 Hell's Circuit

Once in a while the moon turns red, the sky turns dark and there's a green glowing mist rising from the ground and that's exactly how you begin to perceive the world as you get past the 4-minute mark of the first set of Hell's Circuit. Designed to test the mettle of mortals, this a workout that transforms everyone who does it, even at Level I. The exercises appear deceptively easy but don't be fooled. Those who embark upon this little workout without feeling at least a little trepidation are destined for greatness.

Extra Credit: 30 seconds rest between sets.

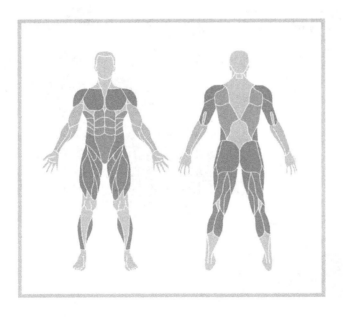

Difficulty

Hell's Circuit

DAREBEE HIIT WORKOUT © darebee.com

Level I 3 sets **Level II** 5 sets **Level III** 7 sets | 2 minutes rest

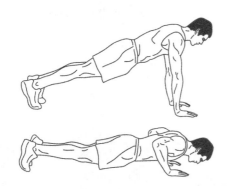

1min push-ups

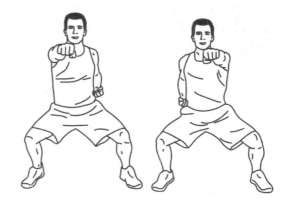

1min squat hold punches

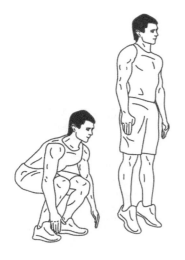

1min jump squats

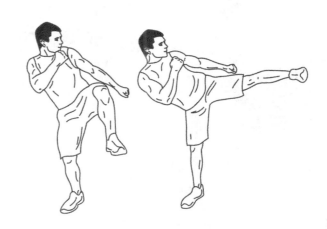

1min side kicks

46 Heyday

Heyday is a Level IV workout that uses both concentric and eccentric muscle movements to challenge the body's VO2 Max limits and raise the body's temperature along with its endurance level. The emphasis here is on speed. You want to get as many reps done in each exercise as possible. Change sides halfway in the kicks and punches for a more balanced muscle and coordination development. When doing crunches it's important to keep your hands by the side of your head but do not hold it. Go for EC and it really gets very tough, very quickly.

Extra Credit: 1 minute rest between sets.

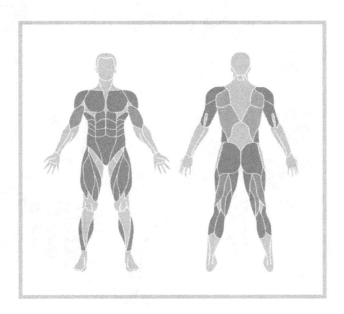

Difficulty

HEYDAY

DAREBEE HIIT WORKOUT © darebee.com

Level I 3 sets **Level II** 5 sets **Level III** 7 sets | 2 minutes rest

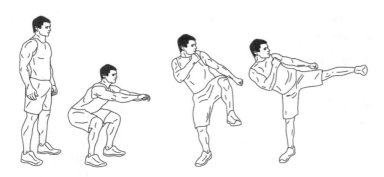

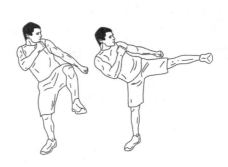

20sec squat + side kicks

40sec side kicks

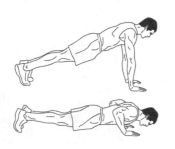

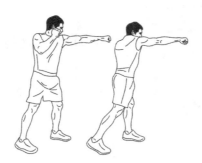

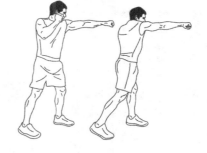

20sec push-up + punches

40sec punches

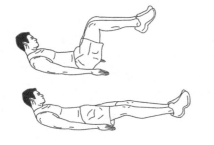

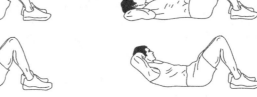

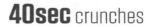

20sec crunch kick + crunch

40sec crunches

47 Homemade Hero

In Homemade Hero you rest by training your core, which means that during the more active part of this HIIT workout you really need to up the intensity and get the numbers in, even if it means reducing the quality of your form. The benefits are stronger, leaner muscles and an aerobic system that will let you catch the bus every time you run for it.

Extra Credit: 1 minute rest between sets.

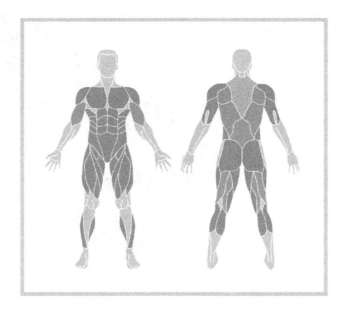

Difficulty

HOMEMADE HERO

DAREBEE HIIT WORKOUT
© darebee.com

Level I 3 sets
Level II 5 sets
Level III 7 sets
2 minutes rest

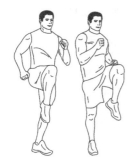

20sec high knees

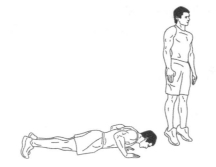

20sec burpees

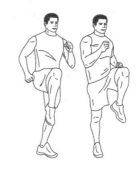

20sec high knees

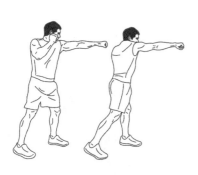

20sec punches

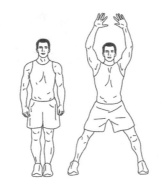

20sec jumping jacks

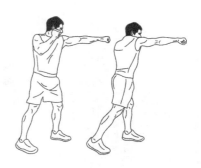

20sec punches

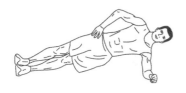

20sec side plank (right)

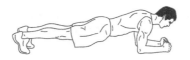

20sec elbow plank

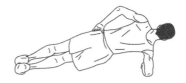

20sec side plank (left)

48 Hotfoot

Hotfoot may look easy but the moment you realize that your knees have to come up to waist height all the time you realize that it will also place a heavy load on your lungs. It certainly does just that. Twist your body when you do march twists and make your you are on the balls of your feet at all times and this is a workout that will seriously challenge you.

Extra Credit: 1 minute rest between sets.

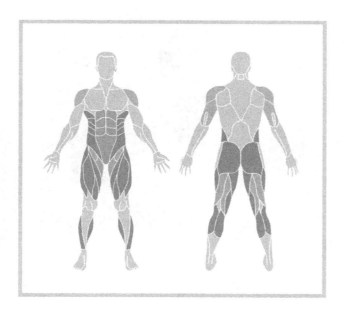

Difficulty

hotfoot

DAREBEE HIIT WORKOUT © darebee.com

Level I 3 sets **Level II** 5 sets **Level III** 7 sets | 2 minutes rest

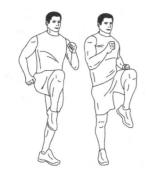

30sec high knees

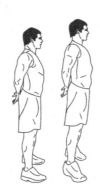

10sec calf raises

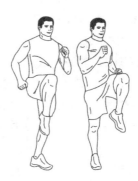

30sec high knees

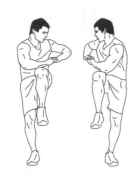

10sec march twists

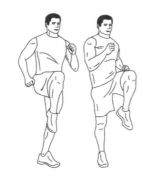

30sec high knees

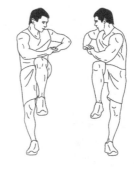

10sec march twists

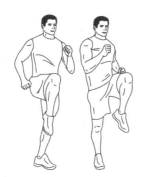

30sec high knees

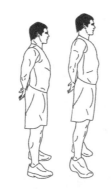

10sec calf raises

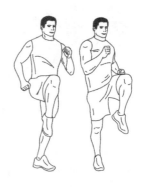

30sec high knees

49 Howler

Some workouts you are prepared for right from the moment you see them and others kinda sneak up on you and leave you feeling wasted on the floor, wondering why you did not see them coming. Howler is definitely one of the latter. Its Level III workout status is deceptive. Bring your knees up to your waist every time you do High Knees, make sure you land on the ball of the foot each time, pump your arms as you run and go as fast as possible in 40 seconds and you realize that this could easily be a Level IV or Level V workout, especially if you add EC.

Extra Credit: Hold the plank in between high knees every time.

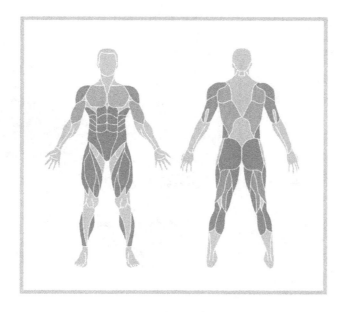

Difficulty

HOWLER

DAREBEE HIIT WORKOUT © darebee.com
LEVEL I 3 sets LEVEL II 5 sets LEVEL III 7 sets REST up to 2 minutes

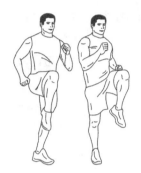

40sec high knees

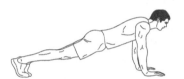

10sec plank

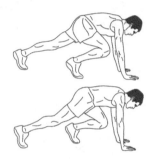

10sec climbers

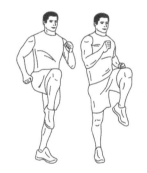

40sec high knees

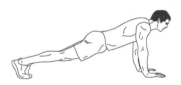

10sec plank

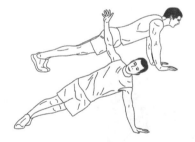

10sec plank rotations

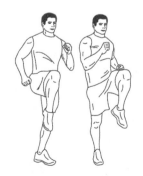

40sec high knees

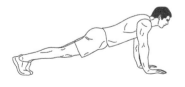

10sec plank

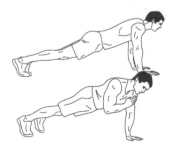

10sec shoulder taps

50 Huff & Puff

When it comes to HIIT speed and rep count are important because they help maintain intensity and it's intensity that delivers results. So, really, for Huff & Puff as for all of the High Intensity Interval Training workouts you want to start as fast and hard as you can, improve on it after the first set or two and then maintain the intensity by keeping track of the rep count for each exercise. That way you're really pushing against the edges of your ability and forcing your body to improve.

Extra Credit: 1 minute rest between sets.

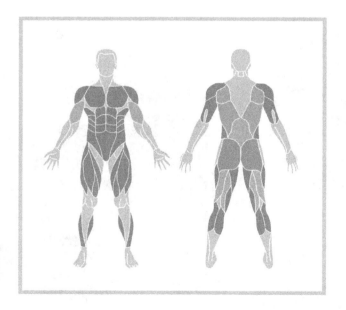

Difficulty

HUFF & PUFF

DAREBEE HIIT WORKOUT © darebee.com

Level I 3 sets **Level II** 5 sets **Level III** 7 sets | 2 minutes rest

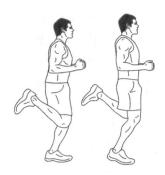

20sec butt kicks

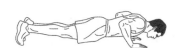

20sec push-up plank hold

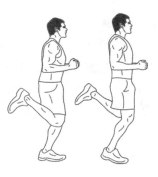

20sec butt kicks

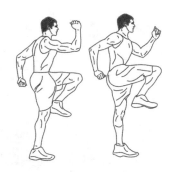

20sec march steps

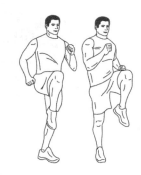

20sec high knees

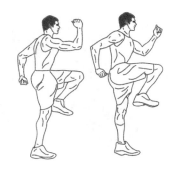

20sec march steps

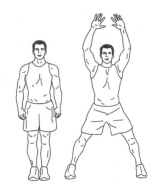

20sec jumping jacks

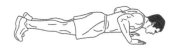

20sec push-up plank hold

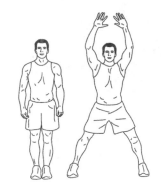

20sec jumping jacks

51 Incinerator

Incinerator is a high-impact aerobic workout that will help you get faster and increase your endurance. High Knees means High Knees here (knees coming up to waist height each time) and you need to pump your arms in order to maintain the pace. Remember to land, always, on the ball of the foot so your heels never touch down. The transition from one exercise to the next should be done as fast as possible and reps really count here so go for as high a number as you can.

Extra Credit: Hit the same number of push-ups every time.

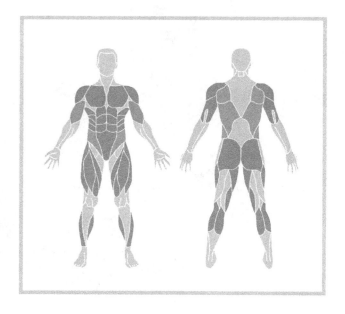

Difficulty

INCINERATOR

DAREBEE HIIT WORKOUT © darebee.com

Level I 3 sets **Level II** 5 sets **Level III** 7 sets **REST** up to 2 minutes rest

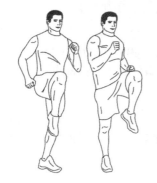

30sec high knees

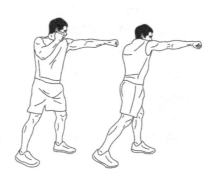

30sec punches

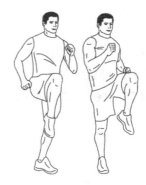

30sec high knees

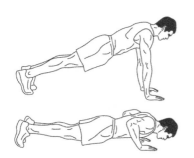

10sec push-ups

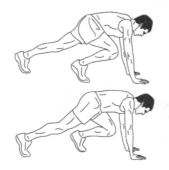

10sec climbers

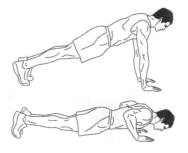

10sec push-ups

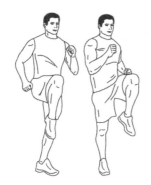

30sec high knees

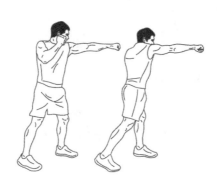

30sec punches

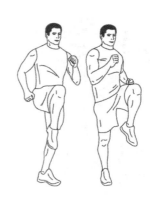

30sec high knees

52   **Inferno**

Inferno is a Level 4 High Intensity Interval Training (HIIT) that places quite the load on the entire body and keeps it there for the duration of the workout. Make sure High Knees are performed by bringing the knee to the height of the waist and keep your body straight and your arms pumping while you are doing it. This is a high-burn, lots-of-sweat kind fo workout so be prepared to feel its effects.

Extra Credit: Hit the same number of burpees in 20 seconds every time.

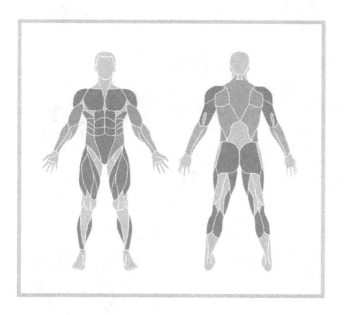

Difficulty

Inferno

DAREBEE HIIT WORKOUT © darebee.com

Level I 3 sets **Level II** 5 sets **Level III** 7 sets **REST** up to 2 minutes rest

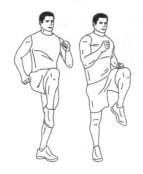 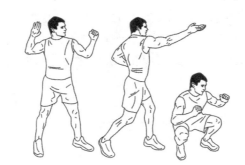 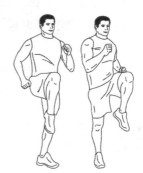

20sec high knees   **20sec** knife hand strike + squat   **20sec** high knees

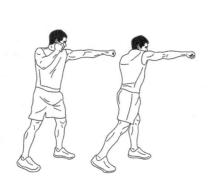 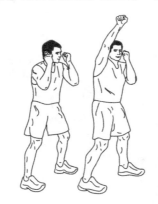 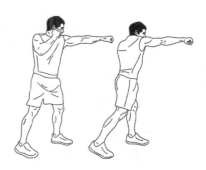

20sec punches   **20sec** overhead punches   **20sec** punches

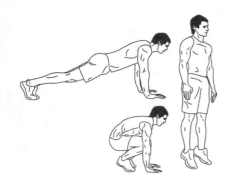 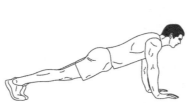 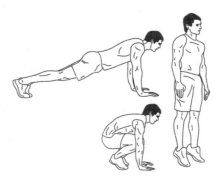

20sec basic burpees   **20sec** plank hold   **20sec** basic burpees

53 Intervention

Intervention will make you stronger, fitter, faster and, according to the latest research, younger at a cellular level. To reap all these benefits you need to pile up the reps and then maintain your focus so that your rep count each time doesn't drop below the number you clock up in your first set (though it can rise if you want). Add EC and you will be even stronger, faster, smarter, younger.

Extra Credit: 1 minute rest between sets.

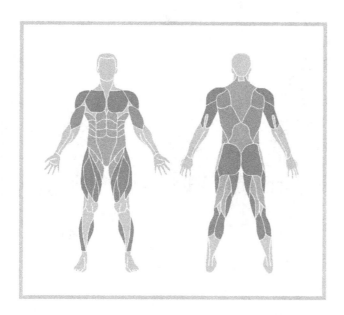

Difficulty

INTERVENTION

DAREBEE `HIIT` WORKOUT © darebee.com

Level I 3 sets **Level II** 5 sets **Level III** 7 sets | 2 minutes rest

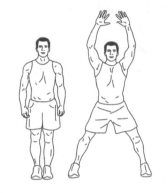

20sec jumping jacks

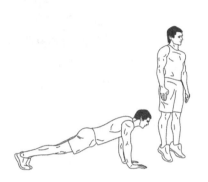

20sec basic burpees

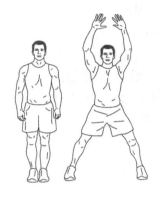

20sec jumping jacks

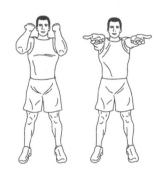

20sec bicep extensions

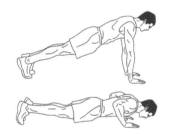

20sec push-ups

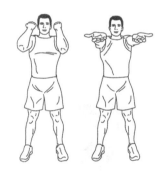

20sec bicep extensions

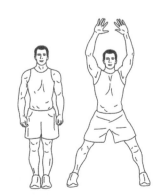

20sec jumping jacks

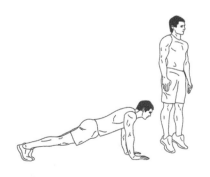

20sec basic burpees

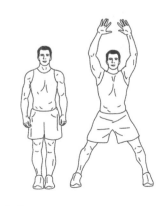

20sec jumping jacks

54   Into The Fire

Combining a number of gravity-fighting moves and combat moves Into The Fire is a workout designed to challenge strength, endurance and coordination. This is a difficulty Level IV workout which means it's not really suitable for those who are new to fitness or for those coming back in from a long lay-off, but it should definitely be on your horizon.

Extra Credit: 1 minute rest between sets.

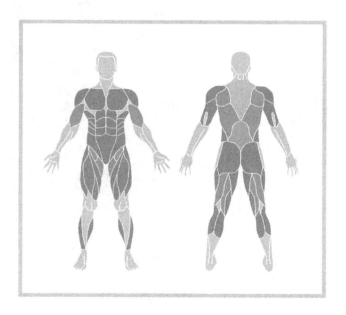

Difficulty

INTO THE FIRE

DAREBEE `HIIT` WORKOUT © darebee.com

Level I 3 sets **Level II** 5 sets **Level III** 7 sets | 2 minutes rest

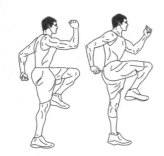

30sec march steps

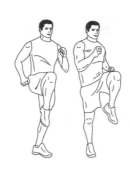

15sec high knees

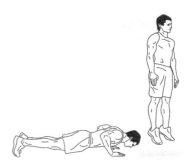

15sec burpees

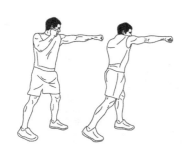

30sec punches

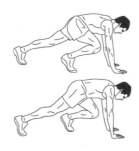

15sec climbers

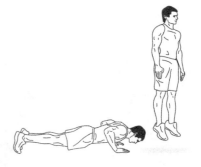

15sec burpees

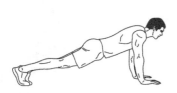

30sec plank hold

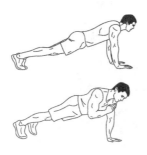

15sec shoulder taps

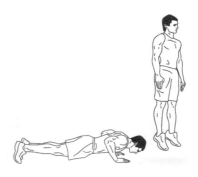

15sec burpees

55   **Mass Blast**

Developed to help you storm hills and race up mountains this is the workout for those looking to unlock all the power of their lower body.

Extra Credit: 30 seconds rest between sets.

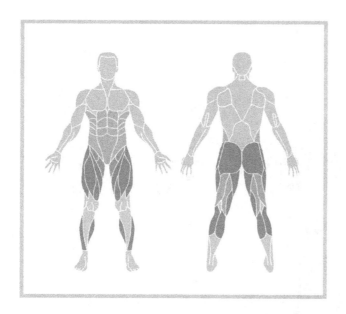

Difficulty

MASS BLAST

DAREBEE HIIT WORKOUT © darebee.com

Level I 3 sets **Level II** 5 sets **Level III** 7 sets | 2 minutes rest

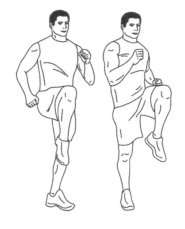

15sec high knees

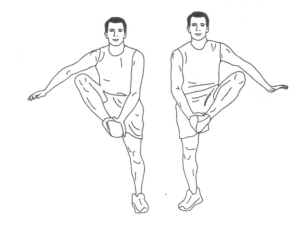

15sec toe tap hops

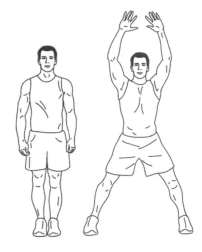

15sec jumping jacks

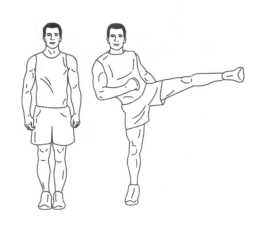

15sec side leg raises

56　Max Impact

Some workouts are designed to deliver at a high-impact, no-holds barred level. If you're ready to take your body to that extra-fit level then this is the one to do.

Extra Credit: 30 seconds rest between sets.

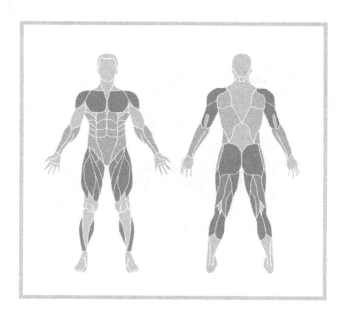

Difficulty

MAX IMPACT

DAREBEE HIIT WORKOUT © darebee.com

Level I 3 sets **Level II** 5 sets **Level III** 7 sets | 2 minutes rest

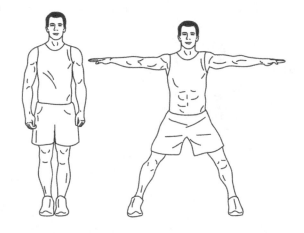

20sec jumping Ts

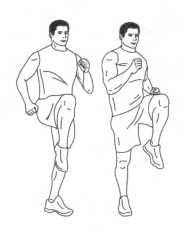

20sec high knees

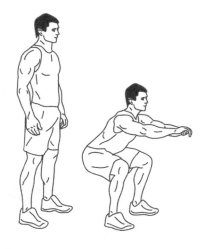

10sec squats

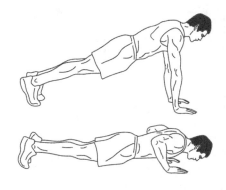

10sec push-ups

57 Max Out

Max Out is a difficulty Level IV workout that loads your lungs by moving large muscle groups all the time and it keeps on loading them as you go from one exercise to another and one set to the next. Form is crucial here, despite the need for a high rep count. Use both arms and legs in coordination in March Steps and High Knees. Go as high as you can as you jump during Burpees.

Extra Credit: 1 minute rest between sets.

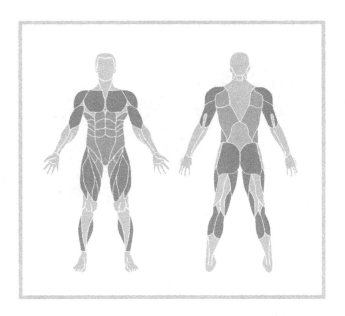

Difficulty

MAX OUT

HIIT WORKOUT
BY DAREBEE
© darebee.com
Level I 3 sets
Level II 5 sets
Level III 7 sets
2 minutes rest

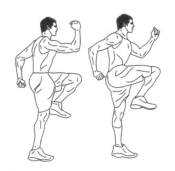

20sec march steps

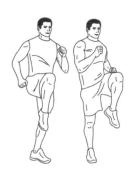

20sec high knees

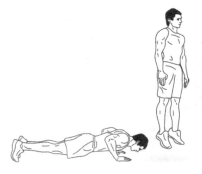

20sec burpees

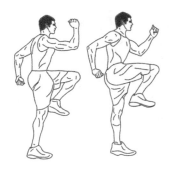

20sec march steps

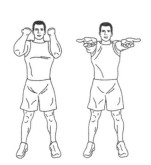

20sec bicep extensions

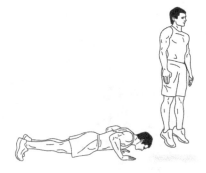

20sec burpees

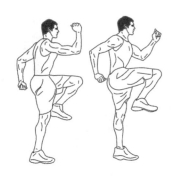

20sec march steps

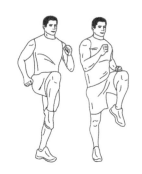

20sec high knees

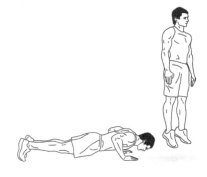

20sec burpees

58 Melt Off

Melt Off uses large muscle groups under a heavy load to test your VO2 Max. Form and rep count are important here. Bring your knees to waist height during High Knees and work fast and hard with your Burpees to get in as many as you can in each 20 second time slot. Your active recovery is the Elbow Plank so breathe slow and deep during those times to oxygenate your muscles. Add EC and the load becomes interesting.

Extra Credit: 1 minute rest between sets.

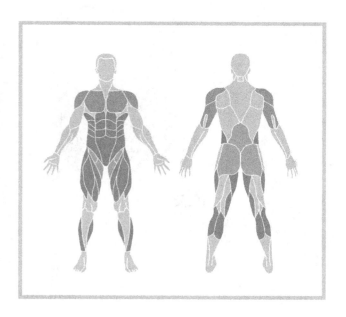

Difficulty

MELT OFF

DAREBEE `HIIT` WORKOUT © darebee.com

Level I 3 sets **Level II** 5 sets **Level III** 7 sets | 2 minutes rest

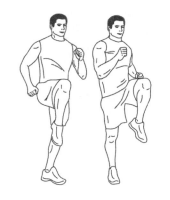

20sec high knees

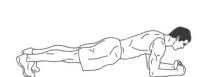

20sec elbow plank

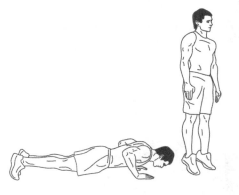

20sec burpees

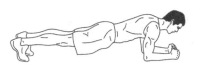

20sec elbow plank

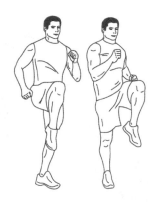

20sec high knees

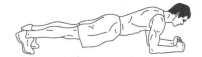

20sec elbow plank

59 New Beginning

The beauty of HIIT is that everyone can do it at their own level, whatever it might be. As long as we give it our all we will see results. HIIT it with the New Beginnings Workout and get back into it, like you mean it. Keep the plank when transitioning from the plank to climbers, plank jacks and plank leg raises, DDD = don't drop down. Go flat out when performing high knees, jumping jacks and butt kicks.

Extra Credit: 1 minute rest between sets.

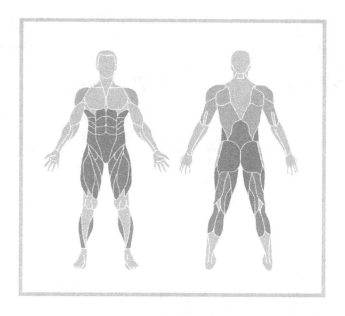

Difficulty

NEW BEGINNING

DAREBEE `HIIT` WORKOUT © darebee.com

Level I 3 sets **Level II** 5 sets **Level III** 7 sets

2 minutes rest

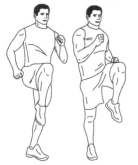

30sec high knees

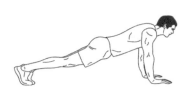

20sec plank hold

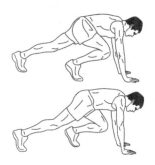

10sec climbers

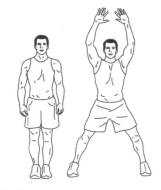

30sec jumping jacks

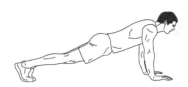

20sec plank hold

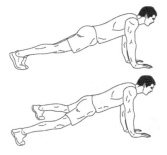

10sec plank jacks

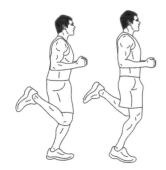

30sec butt kicks

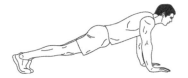

20sec plank hold

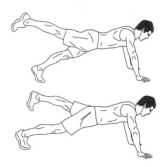

10sec plank leg raises

60 No One Is Watching

Work out like No One is Watching! Because no one probably is. The more variety you have in your routine, the better since your muscles haven't adapted to the new moves and haven't optimized for the minimum energy expenditure required, yet. Go flat out on this one, form is secondary - just have fun with it!

Extra Credit: 1 minute rest between sets.

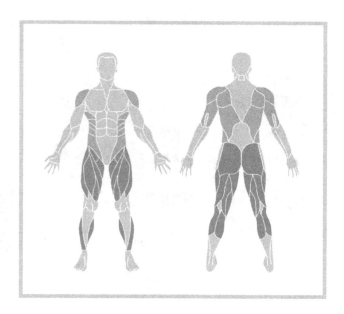

Difficulty

No One is Watching

DAREBEE `HIIT` WORKOUT © darebee.com

Level I 3 sets **Level II** 5 sets **Level III** 7 sets | 2 minutes rest

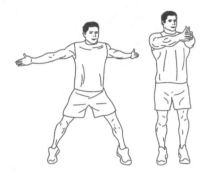

20sec seal jacks

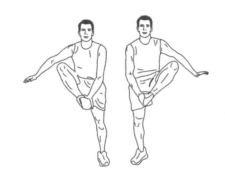

20sec toe tap hops

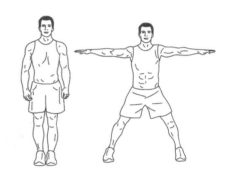

20sec jumping Ts

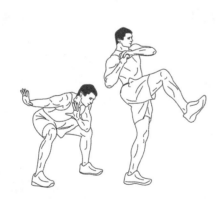

20sec squat step-ups

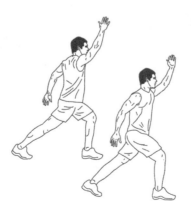

20sec split jacks

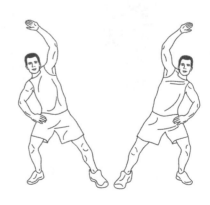

20sec side jacks

61 No Surrender

You know that the moment you get a workout called No Surrender it's really a challenge because surrender is what you'd want to do. Resist the fatigue that's designed to build up and maintain your output throughout each set. This one's all about the intensity and if you like to up the ante just a tad, add EC.

Extra Credit: 1 minute rest between sets.

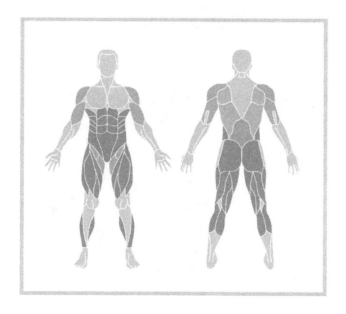

Difficulty

NO SURRENDER

DAREBEE `HIIT` WORKOUT © darebee.com

Level I 3 sets **Level II** 5 sets **Level III** 7 sets | 2 minutes rest

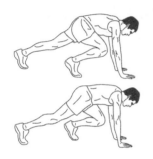

20sec climbers

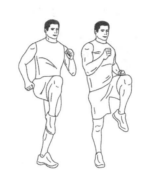

20sec high knees

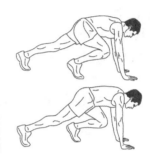

20sec climbers

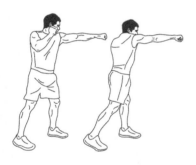

20sec punches

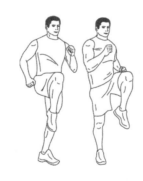

20sec high knees

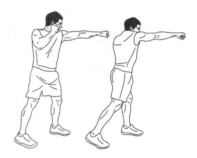

20sec punches

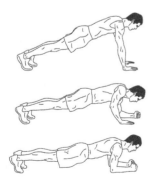

20sec up & down planks

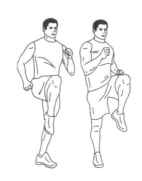

20sec high knees

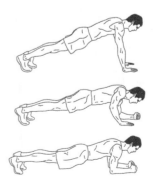

20sec up & down planks

62 Odyssey

The Odyssey took ten years to deliver a result and a lot of personal struggle. Luckily, The Odyssey workout is geared to train you to get there a little bit faster and hard as it may seem, the personal struggle is nothing like its namesake. Add EC, because you know you must and make this one a personal target to conquer.

Extra Credit: 1 minute rest between sets.

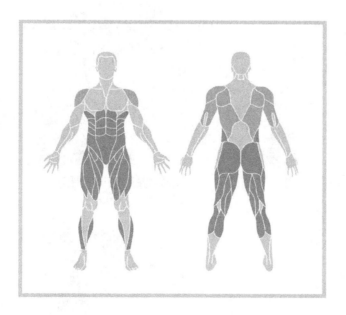

Difficulty

THE ODYSSEY

DAREBEE HIIT WORKOUT © darebee.com

Level I 3 sets **Level II** 5 sets **Level III** 7 sets | 2 minutes rest

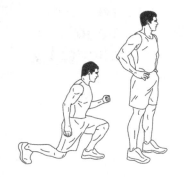

20sec reverse lunges

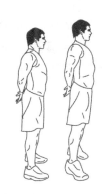

20sec calf raises

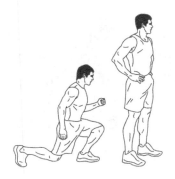

20sec reverse lunges

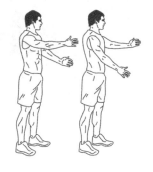

20sec scissor chops

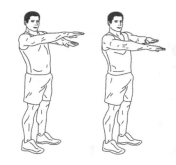

20sec arm scissors

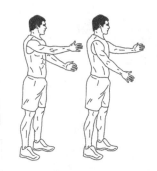

20sec scissor chops

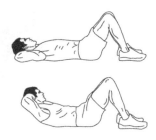

20sec crunches

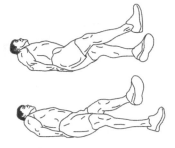

20sec scissors

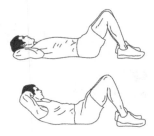

20sec crunches

63 Out Of Excuses

For the days when you want to work hard but don't want to have to think too much the Out Of Excuses workout offers the perfect combination of heavy physical engagement and light mental work. It's a fast, focused workout that will get you sweating very quickly and then will have you breathing hard. The benefits are that as your body works, your mind recharges. You may end up feeling tired but you will definitely want to try and do this again.

Extra Credit: 1 minute rest between sets.

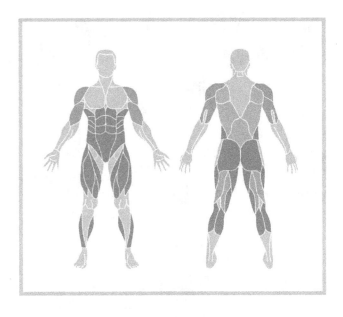

Difficulty

OUT OF EXCUSES

DAREBEE HIIT WORKOUT © darebee.com

Level I 3 sets **Level II** 5 sets **Level III** 7 sets | 2 minutes rest

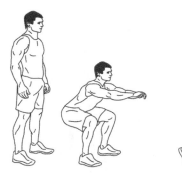

30sec squats

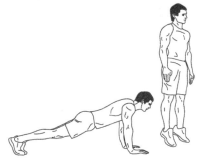

30sec basic burpees

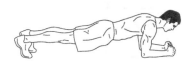

30sec elbow plank

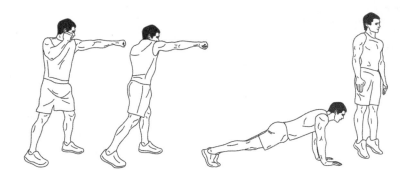

30sec punches

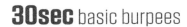

30sec basic burpees

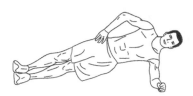

30sec side elbow plank

64 Overdrive

Get your body into overdrive with the Overdrive workout. This is a high intensity Interval Training (HIIT) workout that targets most of the body's major muscle groups. The combination of exercises and combat moves is designed to push your VO2 levels while recruiting secondary muscle groups as fatigue begins to kick in. This will have you in the sweat zone pretty fast and if you add EC you will begin to feel the benefits faster.

Extra Credit: Hit a minimum of 10 reps for every exercises except high knees every time.

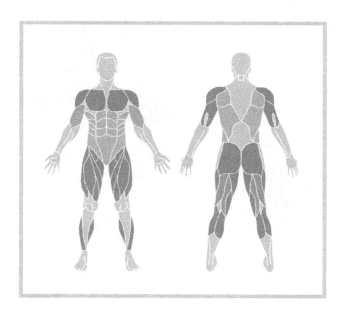

Difficulty

OVERDRIVE

DAREBEE `HIIT` WORKOUT © darebee.com

Level I 3 sets **Level II** 5 sets **Level III** 7 sets **REST** up to 2 minutes rest

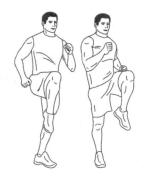

30sec high knees

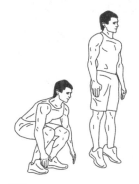

15sec jump squats

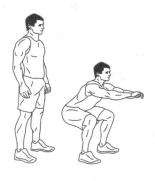

15sec squats

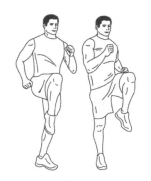

30sec high knees

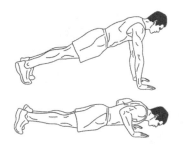

15sec push-ups

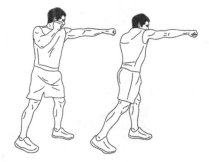

15sec punches

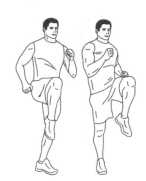

30sec high knees

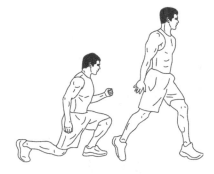

15sec jumping lunges

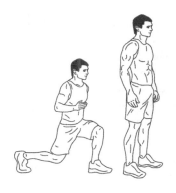

15sec reverse lunges

65   Overhaul

Overhaul is a workout that targets tendons and muscles that power the lower body. It is used to build explosiveness and power. Make sure you bring your knee up to waist-height when performing March Steps and High Knees. Pump your arms in unison with your legs and bring the pace up that way. Try to work to the same count of reps or better each time, throughout each set.

Extra Credit: 1 minute rest between sets.

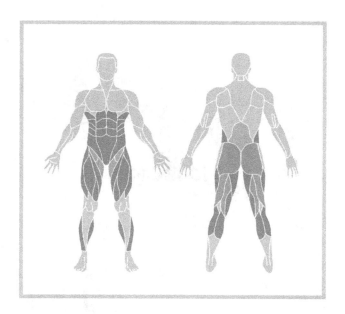

Difficulty

OVERHAUL

DAREBEE `HIIT` WORKOUT © darebee.com

Level I 3 sets **Level II** 5 sets **Level III** 7 sets | 2 minutes rest

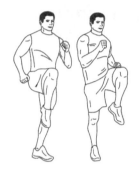
20sec high knees

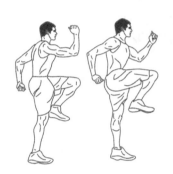
20sec march steps

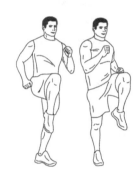
20sec high knees

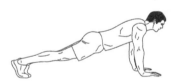
20sec plank hold

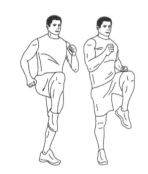
20sec high knees

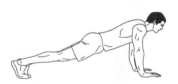
20sec plank hold

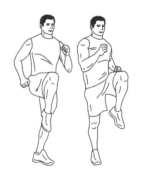
20sec high knees

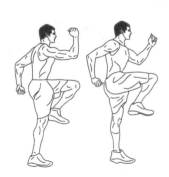
20sec march steps

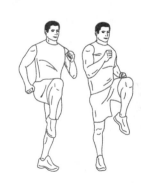
20sec high knees

66 Over The Rainbow

Hyperload your muscles and then try to keep your balance! It's a lot harder than it looks. This workout is not just challenging (and extremely effective), it's also a lot of fun. Take a jump over the rainbow and see how you fair. You can change legs during balance hold halfway through or you can change sides at every set - it's up to you!

Extra Credit: 1 minute rest between sets.

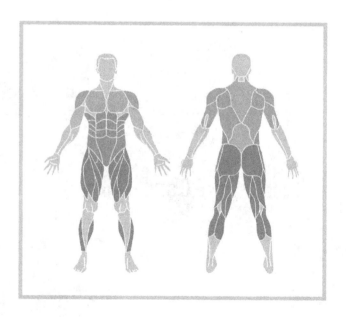

Difficulty

OVER the Rainbow

DAREBEE HIIT WORKOUT © darebee.com

Level I 3 sets **Level II** 5 sets **Level III** 7 sets | 2 minutes rest

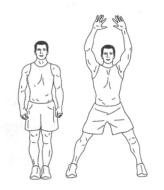

30sec jumping jacks

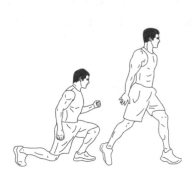

10sec jumping lunges

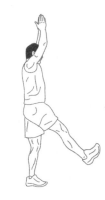

20sec balance hold #1

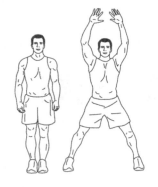

30sec jumping jacks

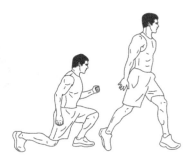

10sec jumping lunges

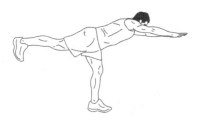

20sec balance hold #2

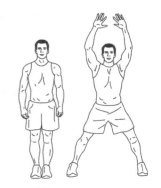

30sec jumping jacks

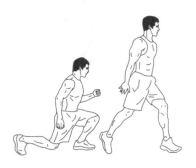

10sec jumping lunges

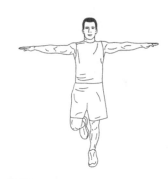

20sec balance hold #3

67 Persephone

Persephone, in Greek mythology, spends half her time in the Underworld and the rest in the world above ground. The workout that bears her name however is all pure Hell Week. Two alternating exercises, performed to perfection, will push your muscles and lungs to the very edge of your capability. This is exactly what you want, right?

Extra Credit: 1 minute rest between sets.

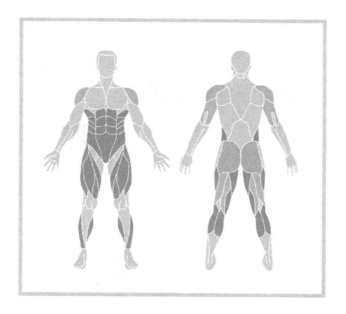

Difficulty

PERSEPHONE

DAREBEE `HIIT` WORKOUT © darebee.com

Level I 3 sets **Level II** 5 sets **Level III** 7 sets | 2 minutes rest

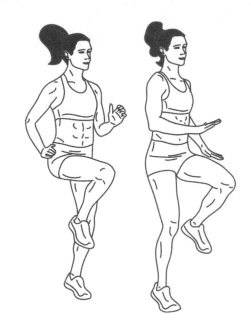

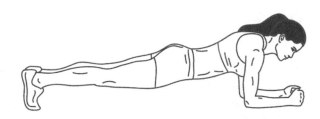

30sec high knees

30sec elbow plank

30sec high knees

30sec elbow plank

30sec high knees

30sec elbow plank

30sec high knees

30sec elbow plank

done

68 Phoenix Burn

The legendary Phoenix rises from its ashes, renewed. Well, this is a little bit like this HIIT workout. Not only will you burn high through it but you will also feel totally renewed once you get to the other side.

Extra Credit: 30 seconds rest between sets.

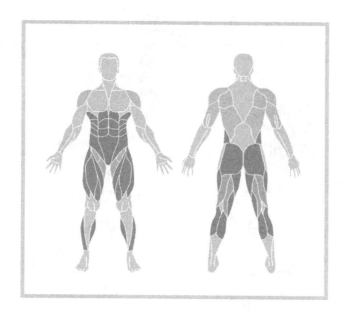

Difficulty

PHOENIX BURN

DAREBEE `HIIT` WORKOUT © darebee.com

Level I 3 sets **Level II** 5 sets **Level III** 7 sets | 2 minutes rest

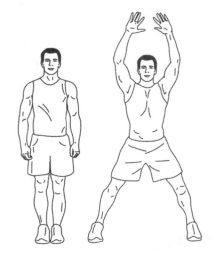

20sec jumping jacks

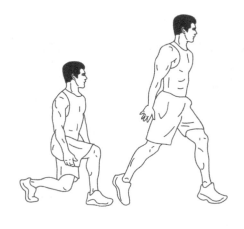

10sec jumping lunges

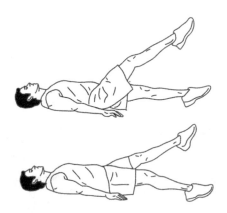

10sec flutter kicks

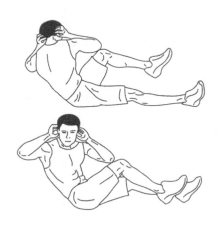

20sec knee-to-elbow crunches

69 Pouncer

The Pouncer workout will work your abs but it won't neglect the rest of your body. It looks deceptively easy and with just two alternating, time-based exercises you'd be tempted to think it is. The Pouncer has a bite however that begins to make itself felt after the first set. Treat with care. Come back to it often.

Extra Credit: 1 minute rest between sets.

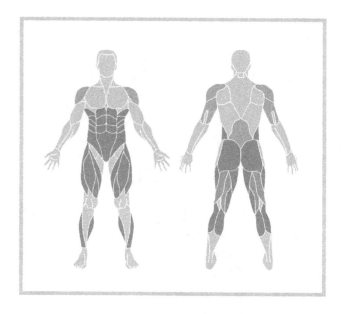

Difficulty

POUNCER

DAREBEE HIIT WORKOUT © darebee.com

Level I 3 sets **Level II** 5 sets **Level III** 7 sets

2 minutes rest between sets

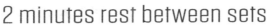
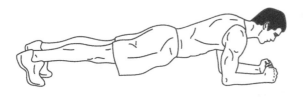
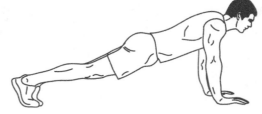

20sec elbow plank

10sec basic burpees

20sec elbow plank

10sec basic burpees

20sec elbow plank

10sec basic burpees

20sec elbow plank

10sec basic burpees

done

70   Power Bolt

It's not the number of exercises you do or even the variety, that matters. It is the intensity and the load they can place on the muscle groups that move the body that make the difference by activating the body's adaptation response. As you're guessing right now, Power Bolt does just that. At less than three minutes per set it uses just two exercises to achieve an almost total body workout. Go high on your Burpees, work really fast with your High Knees, mainatin perfect form throughout and don't forget to land on the ball of the foot, to absorb the impact.

Extra Credit: 1 minute rest between sets.

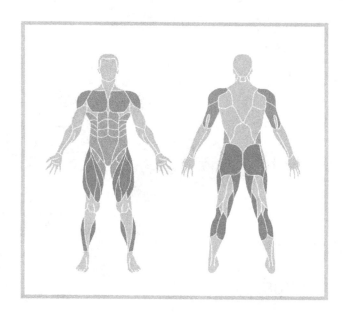

Difficulty

POWER BOLT

DAREBEE `HIIT` WORKOUT © darebee.com

Level I 3 sets **Level II** 5 sets **Level III** 7 sets | 2 minutes rest

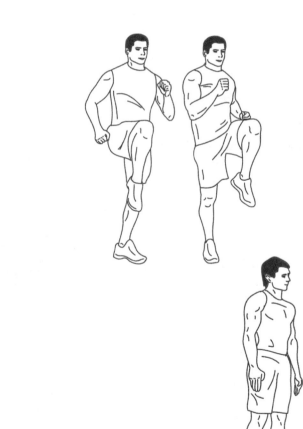

20sec high knees

1 burpee

20sec high knees

1 burpee

20sec high knees

1 burpee

20sec high knees

1 burpee

20sec high knees

1 burpee

20sec high knees

1 burpee

done

71 Power Melt

Power Melt is a high aerobic load workout that will push your lungs to capacity. Pump your arms and bring your knees to waist height during High Knees, go fast on your Burpees and really let rip during your Punches by planting your feet firmly on the floor and using your pelvic muscles to twist your upper body with punches. Go fast on your Push Ups. As you guessed reps really count here and you want to maintain the same number if not go up as you go from set to set. Add EC if all that is not enough.

Extra Credit: 1 minute rest between sets.

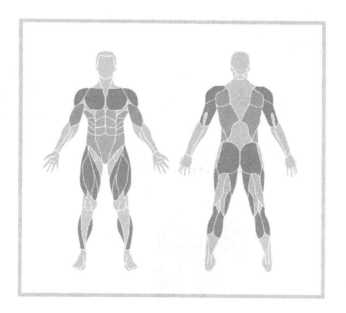

Difficulty

PowerMelt

DAREBEE `HIIT` WORKOUT © darebee.com

Level I 3 sets **Level II** 5 sets **Level III** 7 sets | 2 minutes rest

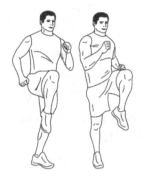

30sec high knees

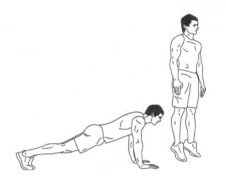

10sec basic burpees

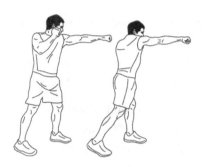

20sec punches

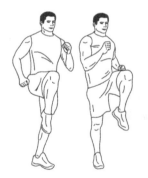

30sec high knees

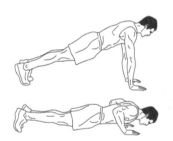

10sec push-ups

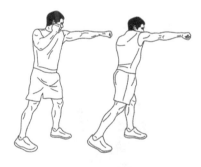

20sec punches

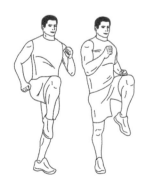

30sec high knees

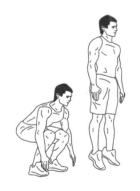

10sec jump squats

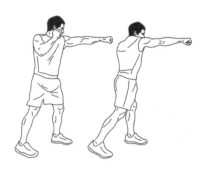

20sec punches

72 **Power Shed**

Power Shed is a fast moving strength and tone workout that also pushes VO2 Max, which means endurance. Each exercise is time-based which means you really need to get the rep count up for each exercise and then aim to keep it there or improve it throughout each set. Get your knees up at High Knees and make sure you're landing on the balls of your feet as you touch down. Plant your feet firmly during punches, left foot forward and then really twist your upper trunk to get body weight behind each punch and snap the punch back fast to get the rep count up. Transition as quickly as you can between exercises, give yourself zero downtime. And add EC. It will make you feel the burn!

Extra Credit: 1 minute rest between sets.

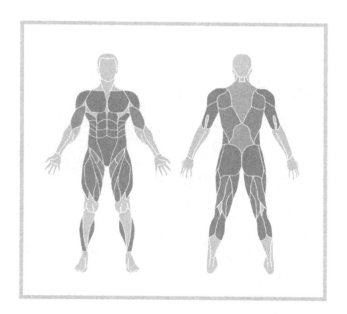

Difficulty

POWER SHED

HIIT WORKOUT
BY DAREBEE
© darebee.com
Level I 3 sets
Level II 5 sets
Level III 7 sets
2 minutes rest

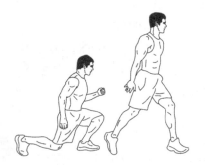
10sec jumping lunges

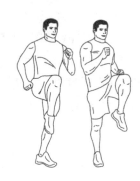
20sec high knees

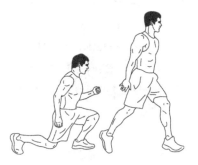
10sec jumping lunges

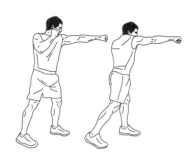
20sec punches

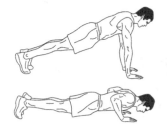
10sec push-ups

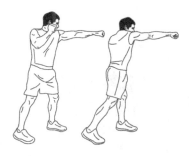
20sec punches

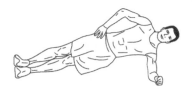
20sec side plank hold

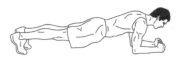
20sec plank hold

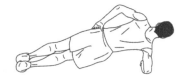
20sec side plank hold

73 Power Strike

Do your body a favor and take it to another performance level entirely with the Power strike workout. This is a fast and furious, HIIT workout that raises the body's temperature, loads the aerobic and cardiovascular systems and pushes every muscle group there is to coordinate and perform better. The constant change from bodyweight to ballistic exercises and back again make sure that the pressure keeps piling up and up and up. You get into the sweat zone from pretty much the first set so you'd better be warmed up properly beforehand. The benefits are strength, speed, power and endurance.

Extra Credit: Keep the number of reps per exercise, per set constant throughout for that extra load, no dipping as you get tired.

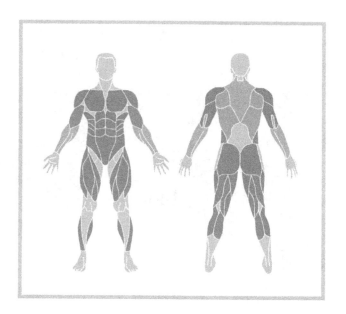

Difficulty

POWER STRIKE

DAREBEE **HIIT** WORKOUT
© darebee.com
LEVEL I 3 sets
LEVEL II 5 sets
LEVEL III 7 sets
2 minutes rest between sets

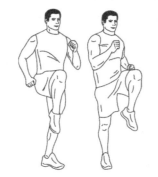 **20sec** high knees

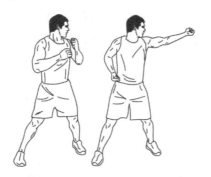 **20sec** backfists

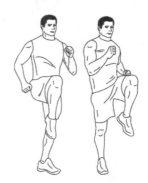 **20sec** high knees

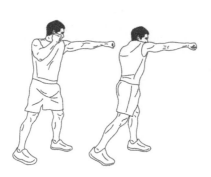 **20sec** punches

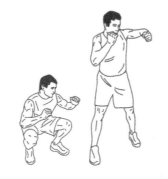 **20sec** squat + hook

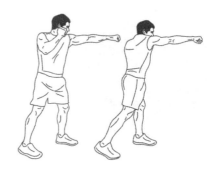 **20sec** punches

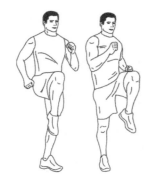 **20sec** high knees

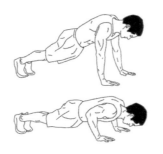 **20sec** push-ups

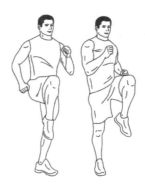 **20sec** high knees

Power Trim

A trim physique is more a function of cumulative exercise, done regularly than the odd hour spent in the gym sweating heavily and using equipment. Make this part of your day and over the course of a year you will see the results.

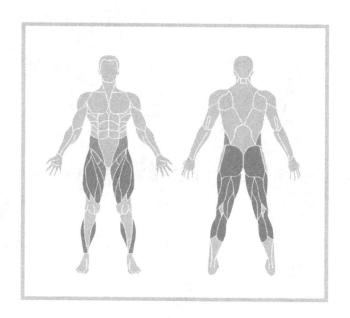

Difficulty

Power Trim

DAREBEE HIIT WORKOUT © darebee.com

Level I 3 sets **Level II** 5 sets **Level III** 7 sets | 2 minutes rest

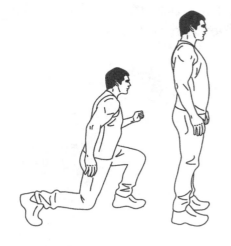

15sec reverse lunges

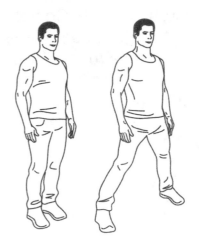

15sec half jacks

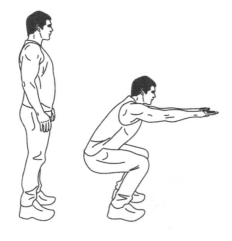

15sec squats

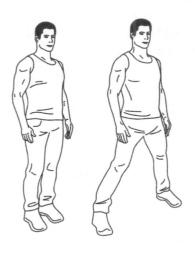

15sec half jacks

75   The Purge

The Purge is a workout that will prepare your body for levelling up. It doesn't just target virtually every major muscle group it also loads them with exercises that demand high intensity. That challenges your VO2 Max and it gets you in the sweatzone quickly. You're kinda getting the implications of this workout's name. Go hard, go fast and bring your knees high on High Knees. Don't forget to be on the balls of your feet throughout the workout, don't let your heels touch down now.

Extra Credit: 1 minute rest between sets.

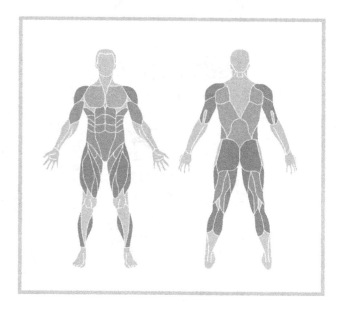

Difficulty

the Purge

HIIT WORKOUT
BY DAREBEE
© darebee.com
Level I 3 sets
Level II 5 sets
Level III 7 sets
2 minutes rest

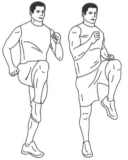

20sec high knees

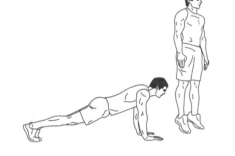

20sec b/burpees w/jump

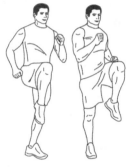

20sec high knees

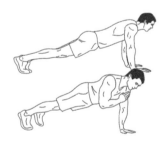

20sec shoulder taps

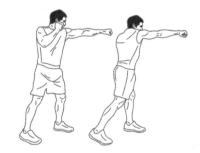

20sec punches

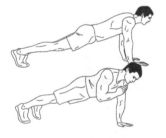

20sec shoulder taps

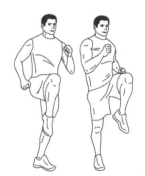

20sec high knees

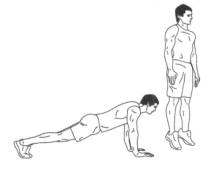

20sec b/burpees w/jump

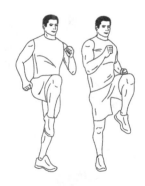

20sec high knees

76 Quick HIIT

Sometimes you just need to HIIT it QUICK! Go flat out, de-stress, take over the world - you can do this! It has it all: cardio, combat, abs and core; all combined in one bad-ass workout. Keep your body straight while holding the plank. Don't drop your arms when transitioning from punches to squat hold punches.

Extra Credit: 1 minute rest between sets.

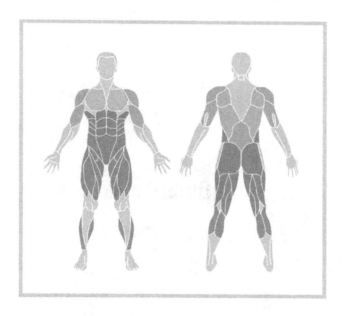

Difficulty

QUICK HIIT

WORKOUT
BY DAREBEE
© darebee.com

Level I 3 sets
Level II 5 sets
Level III 7 sets
2 minutes rest

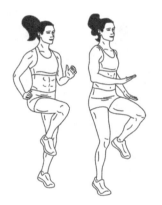

20sec high knees

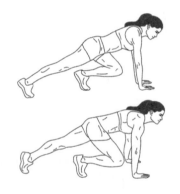

20sec climbers

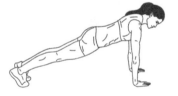

20sec plank hold

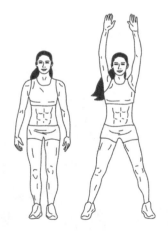

20sec jumping jacks

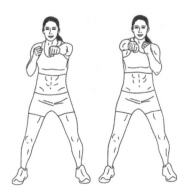

20sec punches

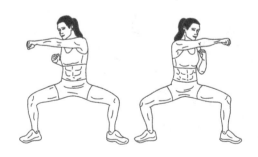

20sec squat hold punches

77 The Rambler

Lower body work utilizes many muscle groups and requires a lot of coordination. It also burns significant amounts of oxygen to power all this. The Rambler is an HIIT workout designed to help you burn hot fast. Go for maximum rep count in each exercise in the allotted time and try to maintain the count throughout each set.

Extra Credit: 1 minute rest between sets.

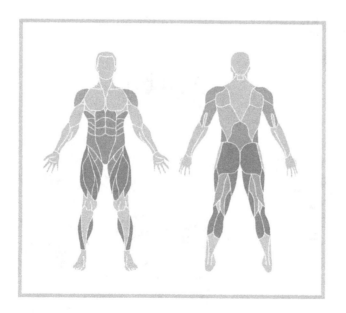

Difficulty

The Rambler

DAREBEE `HIIT` WORKOUT © darebee.com

Level I 3 sets **Level II** 5 sets **Level III** 7 sets | 2 minutes rest

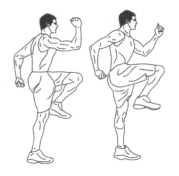

20sec march steps

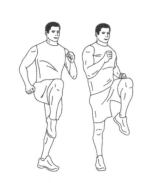

20sec high knees

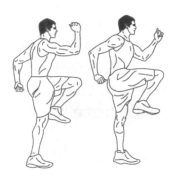

20sec march steps

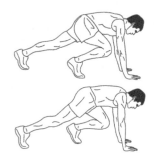

20sec climbers

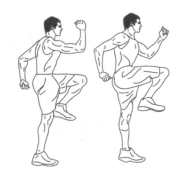

20sec march steps

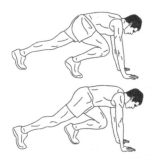

20sec climbers

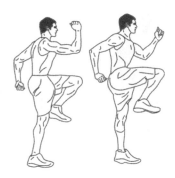

20sec march steps

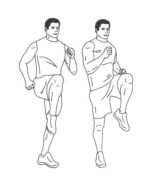

20sec high knees

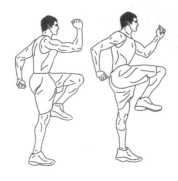

20sec march steps

78 Rapid Fire

Rapid Fire is a fast-paced workout that targets core and abs and demands they work explosively to power the body as you transition from basic Burpees to ground work (Plank) and back again. There are a couple of things to watch out for here in order to get the most out of this workout. First make each transition as fast as possible. Second pack in as many reps as possible in your burpees by moving your legs out and back again to get in burpee jump positions as fast as you can.

Extra Credit: Hit the same number of burpees every time.

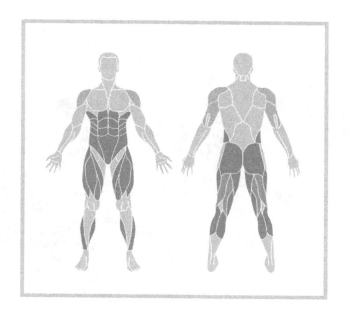

Difficulty

Rapid Fire

DAREBEE `HIIT` WORKOUT © darebee.com

Level I 3 sets **Level II** 5 sets **Level III** 7 sets

2 minutes rest between sets

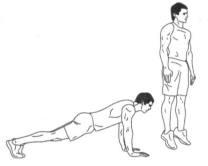

10sec basic burpees

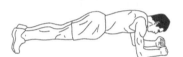

30sec elbow plank

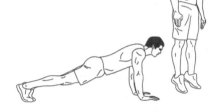

10sec basic burpees

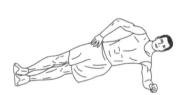

30sec side plank

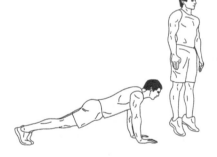

10sec basic burpees

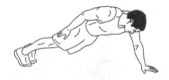

30sec one arm plank

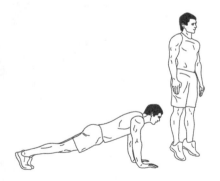

10sec basic burpees

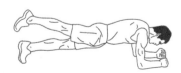

30sec raised leg plank

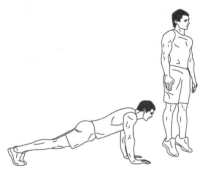

10sec basic burpees

79 Reanimator

Wake up your muscles with a vengeance with the Reanimator workout. Designed to primarily be a lower body workout this one manages to hit all the right notes in quite a lot of secondary muscle groups. While it's suitable for beginners it will still challenge more advanced fitness levels, especially if you add EC.

Extra Credit: 1 minute rest between sets.

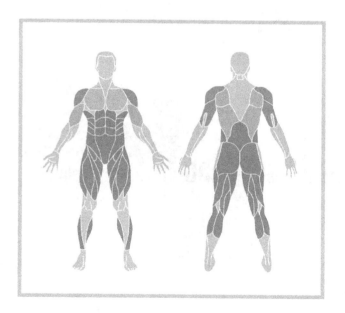

Difficulty

REANIMATOR

DAREBEE `HIIT` WORKOUT © darebee.com

Level I 3 sets **Level II** 5 sets **Level III** 7 sets | 2 minutes rest

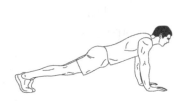

30sec plank hold

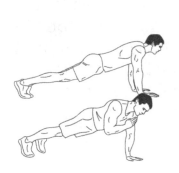

20sec shoulder taps

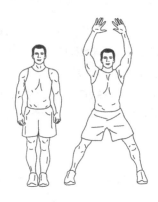

10sec jumping jacks

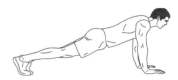

30sec plank hold

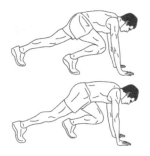

20sec climbers

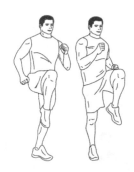

10sec high knees (sprint!)

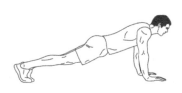

30sec plank hold

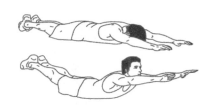

20sec superman stretches

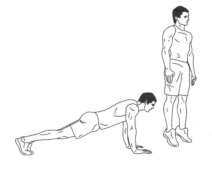

10sec basic burpees

80 **Recalibrator**

Recalibrator is a workout built around Jumping Jacks that form the axis of its routine. This means your form needs to be pitch-perfect. Arms must come up over the side, meet at the very top of your head, in sync with your feet being out and then forcefully brought down, working all arm muscles in both movements. Be on the ball of your feet as you bounce and try and remain on the same count of Jumping Jacks throughout. There are also basic burpees with a jump, but then again you expected that.

Extra Credit: 1 minute rest between sets.

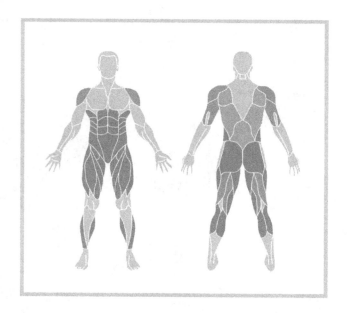

Difficulty

RECALIBRATOR

DAREBEE HIIT WORKOUT © darebee.com

Level I 3 sets **Level II** 5 sets **Level III** 7 sets | 2 minutes rest

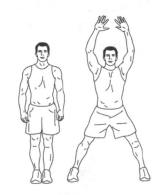

20sec jumping jacks

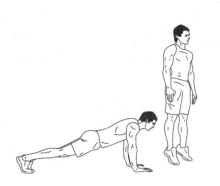

20sec b/ burpees w/jump

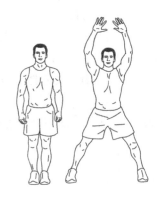

20sec jumping jacks

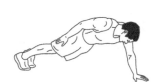

20sec one-arm plank

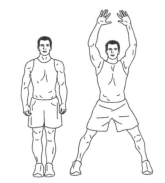

20sec jumping jacks

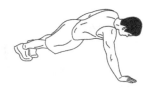

20sec one-arm plank

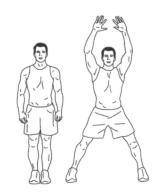

20sec jumping jacks

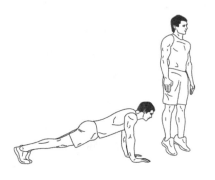

20sec b/ burpees w/jump

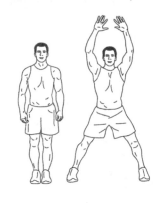

20sec jumping jacks

Reckoning

Combat skills challenge the body and tax the mind The Reckoning offers plenty for both. It's not just the physical side of the exercises. It is also the mental aspect of coordinating each movement, maintaining balance, trying to have perfect form and delivering a smooth, fluid motion. If it all gets a little too much don't worry. It is exactly what it should be.

Extra Credit: 1 minute rest between sets.

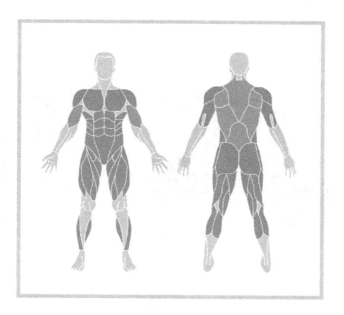

Difficulty

THE RECKONING

DAREBEE `HIIT` WORKOUT © darebee.com

Level I 3 sets **Level II** 5 sets **Level III** 7 sets | 2 minutes rest

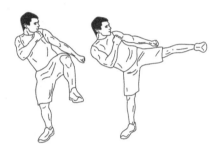

20sec side kicks

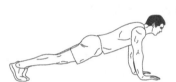

20sec plank hold

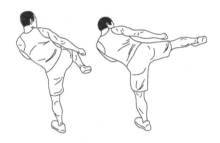

20sec side kicks

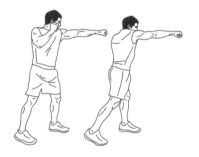

20sec punches

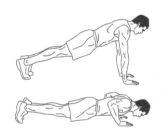

20sec push-ups

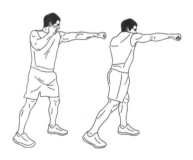

20sec punches

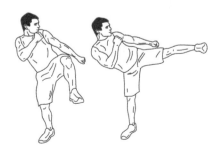

20sec side kicks

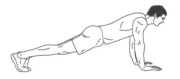

20sec plank hold

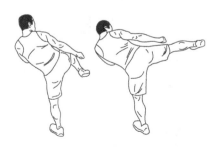

20sec side kicks

82 Rectifier

HIIT exercises up your fitness level, improve VO2 Max and help you get fitter, faster. The Rectifier workout targets your whole body. Like every time-based workout reps and intensity are more important than form so you really want to try and get as many reps in for each exercise as you can and not drop your performance level as you go through the sets.

Extra Credit: 1 minute rest between sets.

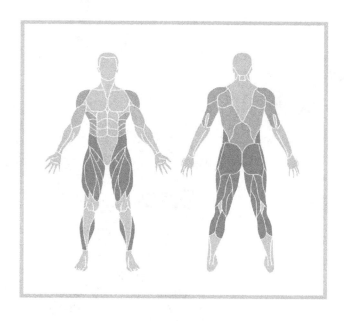

Difficulty

RECTIFIER

DAREBEE HIIT WORKOUT © darebee.com

Level I 3 sets **Level II** 5 sets **Level III** 7 sets | 2 minutes rest

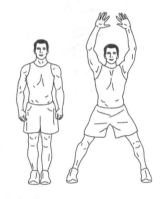

20sec jumping jacks

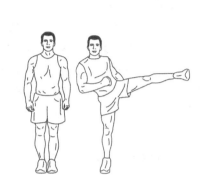

20sec side leg raises

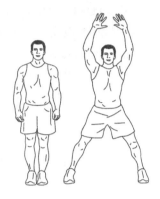

20sec jumping jacks

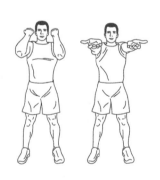

20sec bicep extensions

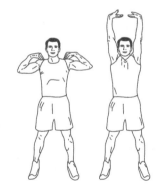

20sec standing shoulder taps

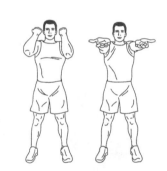

20sec bicep extensions

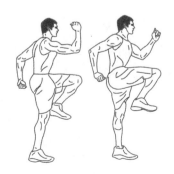

20sec march steps

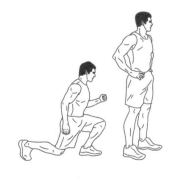

20sec reverse lunges

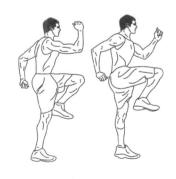

20sec march steps

83 Refiner

When you're looking for a High Intensity Interval Training (HIIT) workout that will help you develop explosive power, endurance, aerobic capability and great recovery time, Refiner should be the one you go to. A difficulty Level IV workout this is not for those new to training and working out, but once you get a little more comfortable with the challenge of pushing your body to perform, this will become a favorite.

Extra Credit: 1 minute rest between sets.

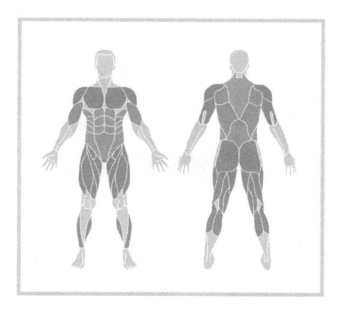

Difficulty

REFINER

DAREBEE `HIIT` WORKOUT © darebee.com

Level I 3 sets **Level II** 5 sets **Level III** 7 sets | 2 minutes rest

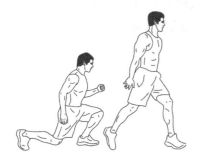

20sec jumping lunges

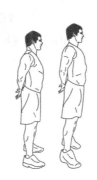

20sec calf raises

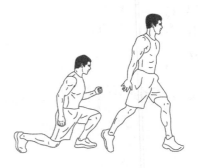

20sec jumping lunges

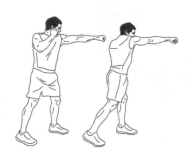

20sec punches

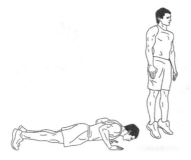

20sec burpees

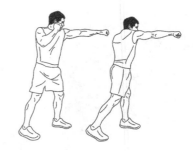

20sec punches

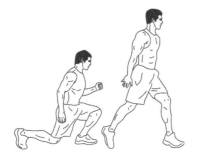

20sec jumping lunges

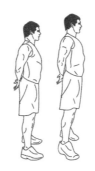

20sec calf raises

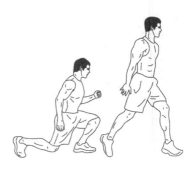

20sec jumping lunges

84 Respawn

The exercise cycle in this workout gives you a hint on why it was named this way. Respawn takes your whole body through a set of exercise that allow each muscle group sufficient time to recover before it is activated fully again. You could potentially do this forever, perfecting it each time you do it.

Extra Credit: 30 seconds rest between sets.

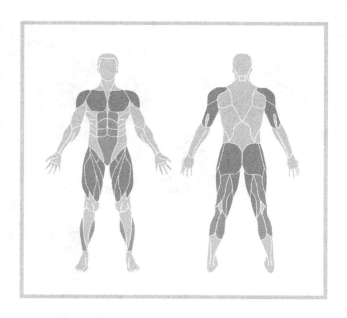

Difficulty

RESPAWN

DAREBEE HIIT WORKOUT © darebee.com

Level I 3 sets **Level II** 5 sets **Level III** 7 sets | 2 minutes rest

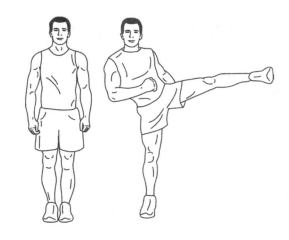

30sec side leg raises

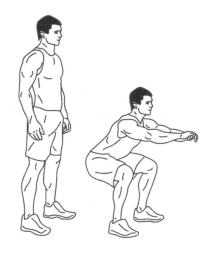

20sec squats

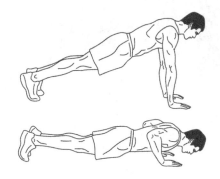

10sec push-ups

85 Reviver

Get back on track with the Reviver Workout. It's an accessible HIIT workout ideal for when you are sore or in recovery but still need an exercise fix. Keep your arms up during bicep extensions and tighten up your core during planks.

Extra Credit: 1 minute rest between sets.

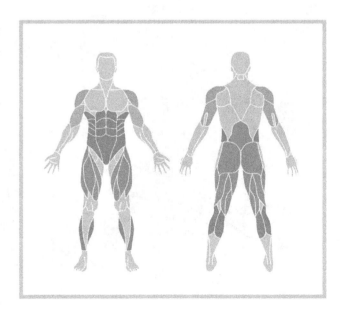

Difficulty

REVIVER

DAREBEE HIIT WORKOUT © darebee.com

Level I 3 sets **Level II** 5 sets **Level III** 7 sets | 2 minutes rest

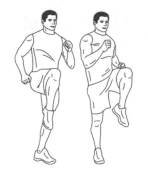

30sec high knees

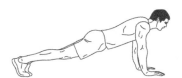

20sec plank hold

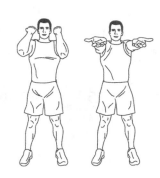

10sec bicep extensions

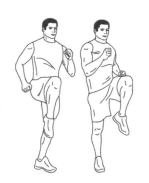

30sec high knees

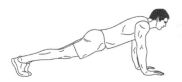

20sec plank hold

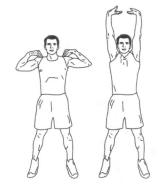

10sec shoulder taps

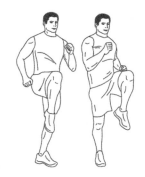

30sec high knees

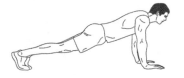

20sec plank hold

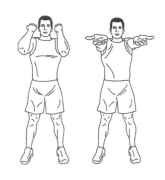

10sec bicep extensions

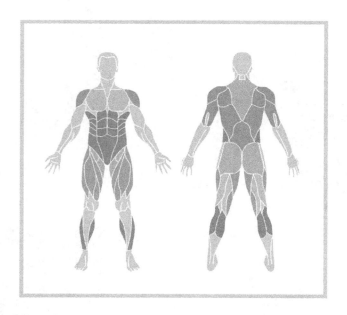

86 Rewired

The Rewired Workout is hard enough to get you working but not too demanding to make you regret it. If you feel it's time to shake off the cobwebs and give your system a full defrag - this is the workout for you. Keep your body straight during planks and go full out during jumping jacks.

Extra Credit: 1 minute rest between sets.

Difficulty

REWIRED

DAREBEE HIIT WORKOUT © darebee.com

Level I 3 sets **Level II** 5 sets **Level III** 7 sets | 2 minutes rest

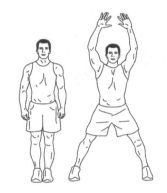

20sec jumping jacks

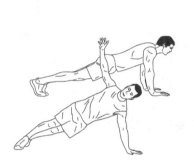

20sec plank rotations

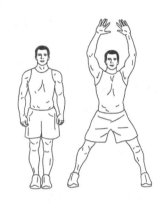

20sec jumping jacks

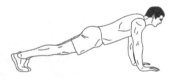

20sec plank hold

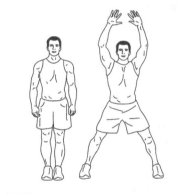

20sec jumping jacks

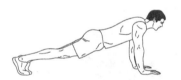

20sec plank hold

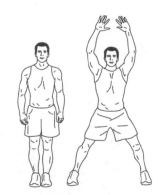

20sec jumping jacks

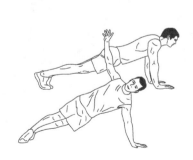

20sec plank rotations

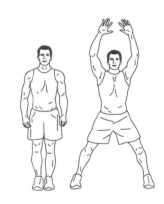

20sec jumping jacks

Ricochet

Combat moves when coupled with callisthenics produce an interesting challenge: muscles have to work ballistically and with resistance which means the dynamic range of motion is challenged both ways. Ricochet provides a workout that will tire you out faster than you expect and will challenge your conditioning. Then again that's what you're here for. Right? Add EC and you're ready to level up.

Extra Credit: 1 minute rest between sets.

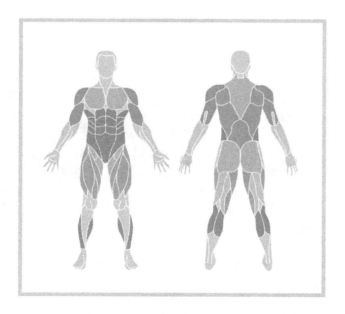

Difficulty

RICOCHET

DAREBEE `HIIT` WORKOUT © darebee.com

Level I 3 sets **Level II** 5 sets **Level III** 7 sets

2 minutes rest between set

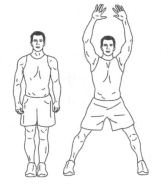

30sec jumping jacks

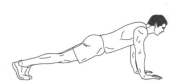

15sec plank hold

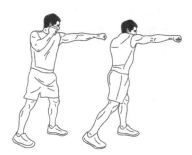

15sec punches

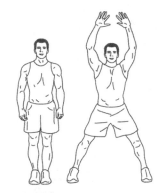

30sec jumping jacks

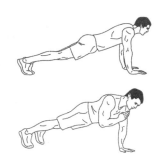

15sec shoulder taps

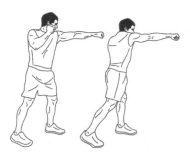

15sec punches

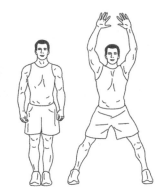

30sec jumping jacks

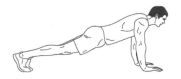

15sec plank hold

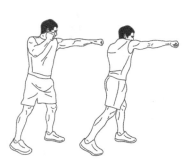

15sec punches

88 Rocket Fuel

High Intensity Interval Training (HIIT) is rocket-fuel to your muscles which is why the Rocket Fuel workout is here to help you reach new performance levels. Because you're always chasing your own performance horizon there is never an easy setting on this, though the difficulty level is subjective. Do it in a half-hearted way and you instantly reduce the benefits it will give you. Go full-out in each 20-second burst and you'll soon feel the burn and the benefits.

Extra Credit: Stay on the balls of your feet throughout. Never let your heels touch down.

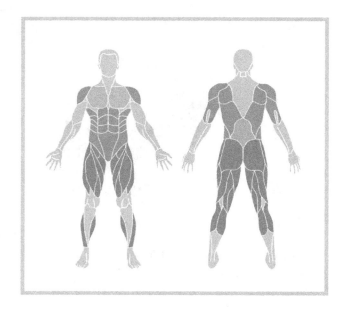

Difficulty

Rocket Fuel

DAREBEE HIIT WORKOUT © darebee.com

Level I 3 sets **Level II** 5 sets **Level III** 7 sets **REST** up to 2 minutes rest

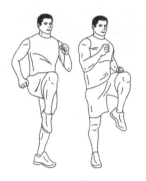

20sec high knees

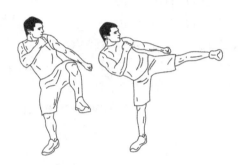

20sec side kicks

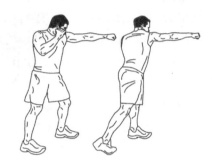

20sec punches

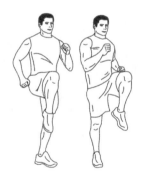

20sec high knees

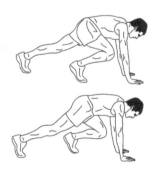

20sec climbers

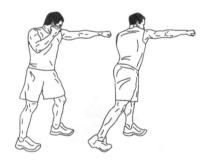

20sec punches

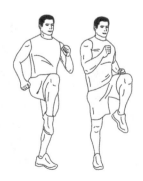

20sec high knees

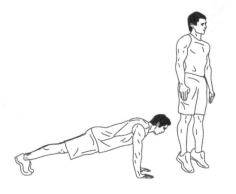

20sec basic burpees

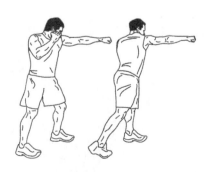

20sec punches

Run & Gun

HIIT workouts are all the rage and Run And Gun doe snot disappoint. It is fast, light, uses every major muscle group there is and gets you in the sweat zone within the first three minutes (set 1). The question after that is just how much can you push yourself so you can improve faster? Can your knees go higher during High Knees? Can you pump your arms more? Can you punch faster? can your hooks be sharper and your upper cuts driven by your bending your knees more? These are questions you get the chance to find the answer to.

Extra Credit: 1 push-up every 20 seconds.

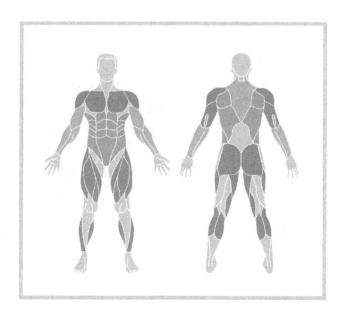

Difficulty

run&gun

DAREBEE **HIIT** WORKOUT © darebee.com

Level I 3 sets **Level II** 5 sets **Level III** 7 sets **REST** up to 2 minutes rest
Extra Credit 1 push-up every 20 seconds

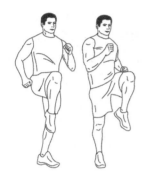
20sec high knees

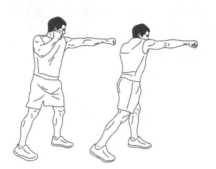
20sec punches

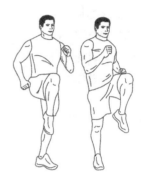
20sec high knees

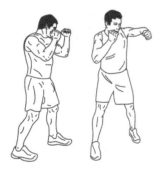
20sec hooks

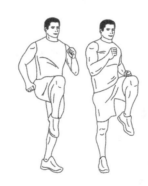
20sec high knees

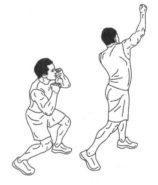
20sec uppercuts

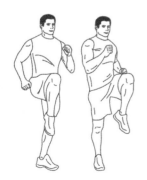
20sec high knees

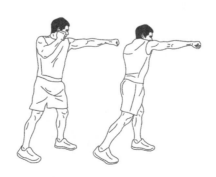
20sec punches

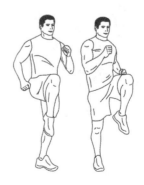
20sec high knees

90 Playing With Scissors

Playing with Scissors is a seemingly easy workout that mirrors upper and lower body tendon/muscle groups load to produce a complete workout that will make you faster and more powerful. Speed in execution is of the essence here. Keep your arms and legs perfectly straight and move them fast. Stay on the balls of your feet throughout Jumping Jacks. You will feel the difference once it's all over.

Extra Credit: 1 minute rest between sets.

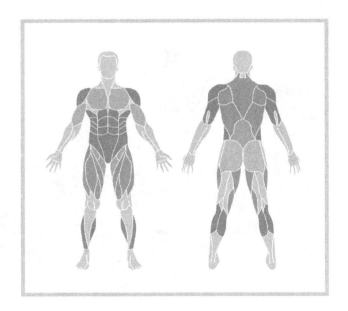

Difficulty

playing with
scissors

DAREBEE `HIIT` WORKOUT © darebee.com

Level I 3 sets **Level II** 5 sets **Level III** 7 sets | 2 minutes rest

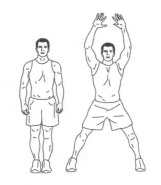

20sec jumping jacks

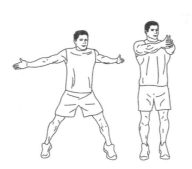

20sec seal jacks

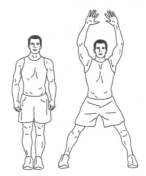

20sec jumping jacks

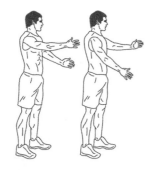

20sec scissor chops

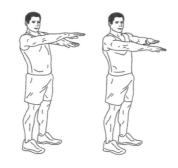

20sec arm scissors

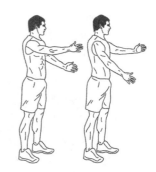

20sec scissor chops

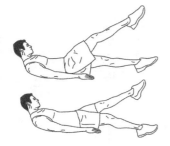

20sec flutter kicks

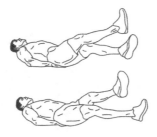

20sec scissors

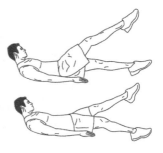

20sec flutter kicks

91 Shifter

Do shifters need to have great freedom of movement to physically morph from one form to another? We don't know for sure. But we do know that if you have the moves then you can walk the walk and talk the talk.

Extra Credit: 30 seconds rest between sets.

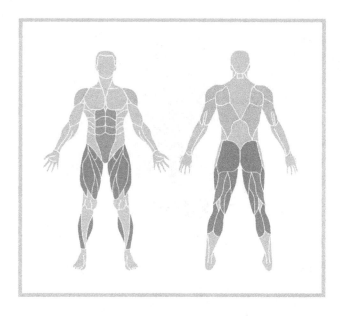

Difficulty

SHIFTER

DAREBEE HIIT WORKOUT © darebee.com
Level I 3 sets Level II 5 sets Level III 7 sets | 2 minutes rest

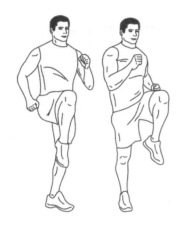

20sec high knees

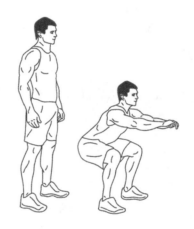

20sec squats

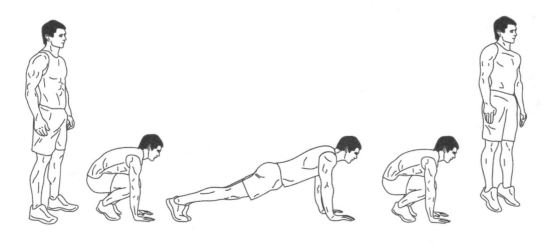

20sec basic burpees

92   **Silver**

The silver workout is a deceptively gentle set of exercises designed to get your body going without too much fanfare or undue pressure on muscle groups. This makes it one of those stealth mode workouts you can do when you're not sure you should be exercising or when you are in recuperative mode, or when simply you're stuck for a workout routine, do not want to wake the neighbours or advertise the fact you're working out. Plus, this is perfect for those just starting out on their journey to personal awesomeness.

Extra Credit: 30 seconds rest between sets.

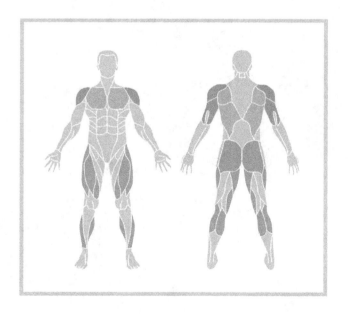

Difficulty

SILVER

DAREBEE `HIIT` WORKOUT © darebee.com

Level I 3 sets **Level II** 5 sets **Level III** 7 sets | 2 minutes rest

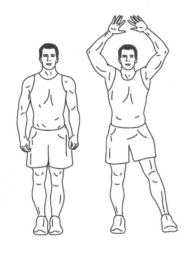

20sec step jacks

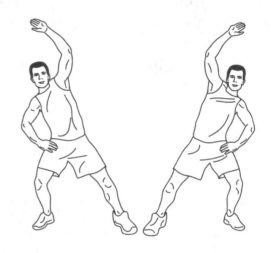

20sec step side jacks

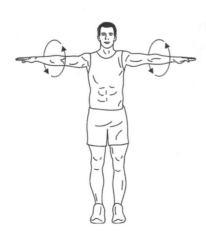

20sec raised arm rotations

93 The Sizzler

The Sizzler is the kind of HIIT workout where you can increase the intensity by adding a little precision to your form. Stay on the balls of your feet throughout, for instance, and insist on bringing your arms down as fast as you send them up during Jumping Jacks and you get a pretty intense HIIT experience that will have you in the sweatzone from the very first set. Add EC and the challenge gets pretty real.

Extra Credit: 1 minute rest between sets.

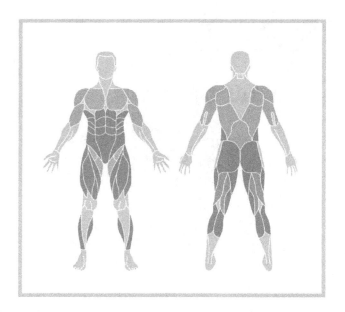

Difficulty

the sizzler

DAREBEE HIIT WORKOUT © darebee.com

Level I 3 sets **Level II** 5 sets **Level III** 7 sets

2 minutes rest between sets

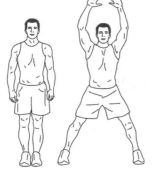

20sec jumping jacks

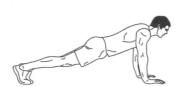

20sec plank hold

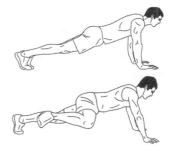

20sec side crunches

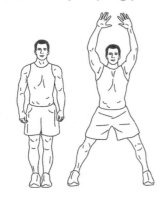

20sec jumping jacks

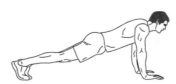

20sec plank hold

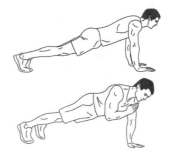

20sec shoulder taps

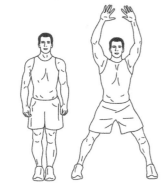

20sec jumping jacks

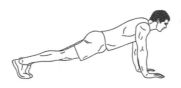

20sec plank hold

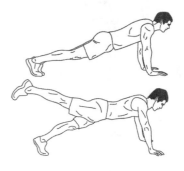

20sec leg raises

94 Skydiver

Skydiver is a full body HIIT workout that utilizes rapid limb movements and coordinated upper/lower body exercises to create a load on practically every major muscle group in the body. You want to maintain form in this one, trying to get the full range of movement where it's required and still get as many reps in as possible. This is a sweat-inducing workout that will get you into the "hot zone" of your performance cycle and keep you there, particularly if you also add EC.

Extra Credit: 1 minute rest between sets.

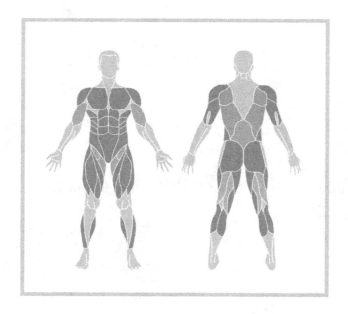

Difficulty

skydiver

DAREBEE HIIT WORKOUT © darebee.com

Level I 3 sets **Level II** 5 sets **Level III** 7 sets | 2 minutes rest

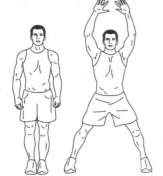

20sec jumping jacks

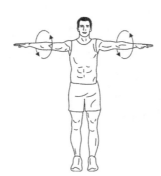

20sec raised arm circles

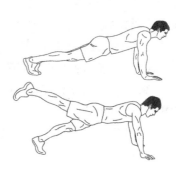

20sec plank leg raises

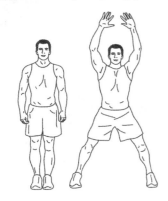

20sec jumping jacks

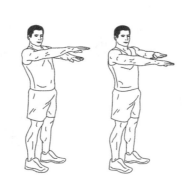

20sec arm scissors

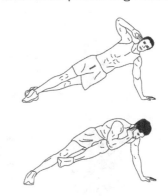

20sec side plank knee-to-elbow

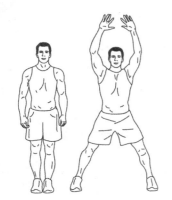

20sec jumping jacks

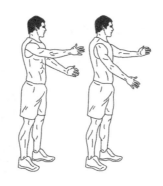

20sec arm chops

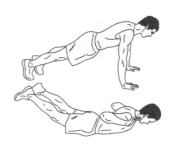

20sec sky diver push-ups

Smoking Hot

This workout is for those who like it hot and are not afraid to go an extra mile for that extra burn. Slightly longer than a traditional DAREBEE HIIT circuit this routine is here to add some spice to your day. To get the most out of your workout keep the plank during the plank to push-up transition and all the way through the final plank sequence. The calf raises are not there for you to rest, make sure you go up and down as fast as can - it's HIIT after all! Keep your arms up during bicep extensions so your elbows point forward for all 40 seconds each time. If you feel the burn, your are on the right track.

Extra Credit: Keep the plank whenever possible.

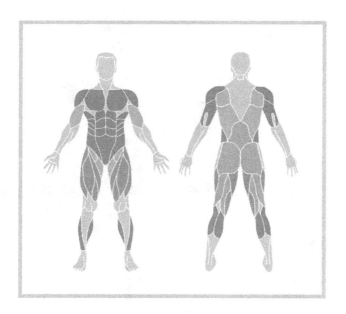

Difficulty

SMOKING HOT

DAREBEE **HIIT** WORKOUT
ⓒ darebee.com

Level I 3 sets **Level II** 5 sets **Level III** 7 sets
2 minutes rest between sets

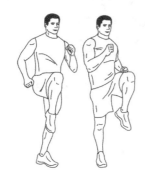

20sec high knees

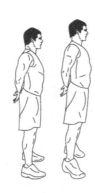

20sec calf raises

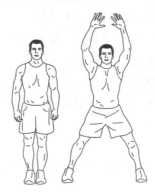

40sec jumping jacks

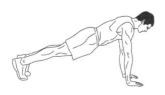

20sec plank hold

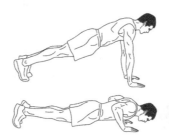

20sec push-ups

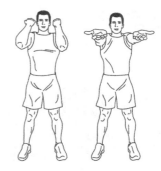

40sec bicep extensions

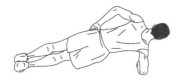

20sec side plank hold
- right -

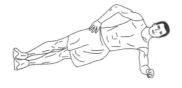

20sec side plank hold
- left -

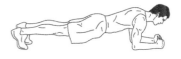

40sec elbow plank hold

96   **SOS**

SOS is a fast-moving, hard-hitting HIIT workout that demands explosion and consistent pressure throughout each set. Stay on your toes throughout your Jumping Jacks routine and make sure you also always land on the ball of the foot after each Jump Knee Tuck. bring your knees to your chest with Jump Knee Tucks and move as explosively as you can within the 10 sec segment of the workout. You will feel the burn and there is always fatigue to battle against. Then again this is the kind of workout you may need rescue from, and that's before you add EC.

Extra Credit: Hit the same number of jump knee tucks every time.

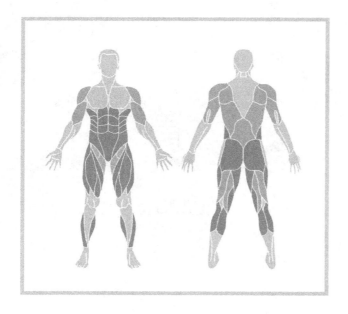

Difficulty

SOS

DAREBEE `HIIT` WORKOUT © darebee.com

Level I 3 sets **Level II** 5 sets **Level III** 7 sets

2 minutes rest

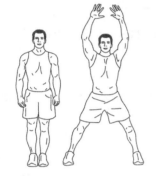

30sec jumping jacks

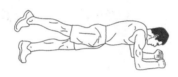

20sec raised leg e/plank

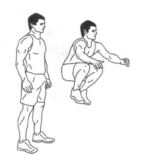

10sec jump knee tucks

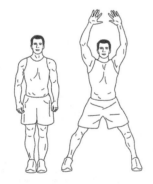

30sec jumping jacks

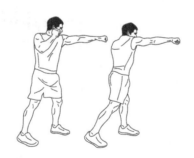

20sec punches

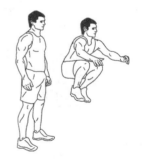

10sec jump knee tucks

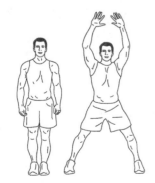

30sec jumping jacks

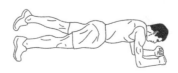

20sec raised leg e/plank

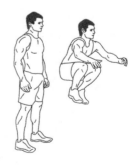

10sec jump knee tucks

97 Super Burn

Get your body into the Super Burn zone with this workout for guaranteed super sweat! Go as fast as you can and try to hit the same number of reps every time you complete each exercise. Keep your arms up throughout the second row of exercises for Extra Credit and aim for a minimum of 10 basic burpees (no push-up) per 20 seconds each time to get the most out of this routine. Catch your breath and repeat!

Extra Credit: Keep arms up at #3, #4 & #5 and do a minimum of 10 basic burpees each time.

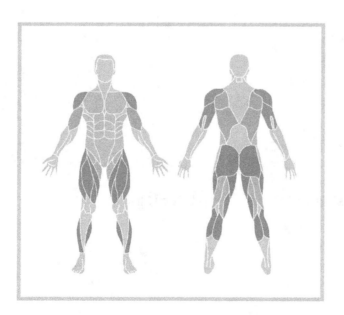

Difficulty

SUPER BURN

DAREBEE HIIT WORKOUT © darebee.com

Level I 3 sets **Level II** 5 sets **Level III** 7 sets | 2 minutes rest

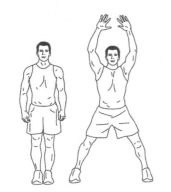

20sec jumping jacks

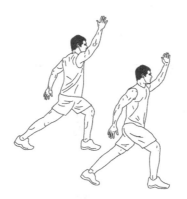

20sec split jacks

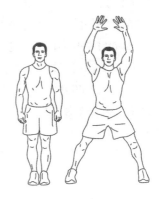

20sec jumping jacks

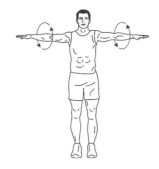

20sec arm circles

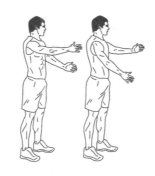

20sec scissor chops

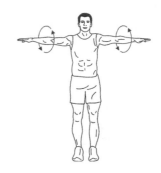

20sec arm circles

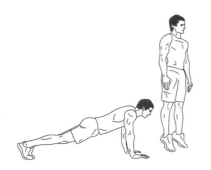

20sec basic burpees

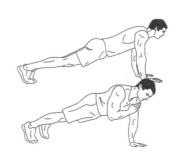

20sec shoulder taps

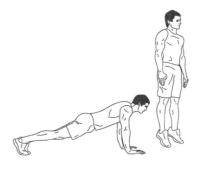

20sec basic burpees

98   Super HIIT

Every now and then you really feel like a "reset" HIIT session, the kind of session that will superheat your muscles, make you sweat hard and leave you feeling totally wiped out afterwards. There are good reasons for sessions like that and they have to do with levelling up. Bring your knees waist high during High Knees, sync your arms and legs, and try to get in as many reps as possible in each 20-second segment. Even done once a month this particular HIIT workout will deliver tangible benefits in overall physical performance.

Extra Credit: 1 minute rest between sets.

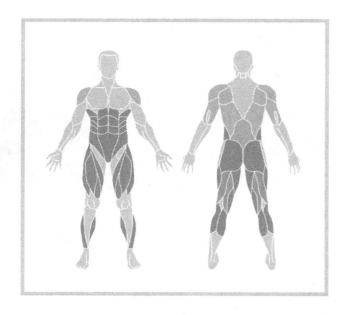

Difficulty

SUPER HIIT

DAREBEE WORKOUT © darebee.com

Level I 3 sets **Level II** 5 sets **Level III** 7 sets | 2 minutes rest

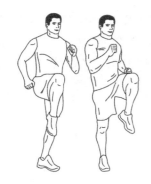

20sec high knees

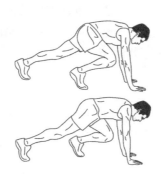

20sec climbers

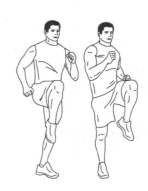

20sec high knees

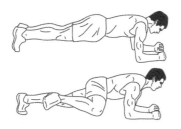

20sec plank crunches

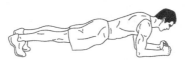

20sec plank hold

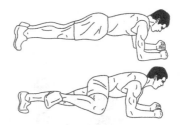

20sec plank crunches

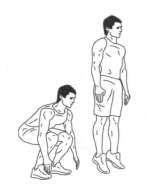

20sec jump squats

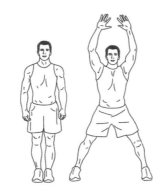

20sec jumping jacks

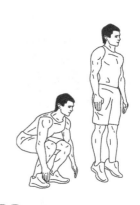

20sec jump squats

Sweat Inc.

Sweat Inc., is not a difficult workout but boy does it target tendons, core, lateral abs and satellite muscle groups (in addition to recruiting some large muscle groups) the way few other workouts do. The result is a challenging workout that lives up to the billing of its name and helps you raise the bar on your athletic performance. Plus it's accessible to practically every level of fitness.

Extra Credit: 1 minute rest between sets.

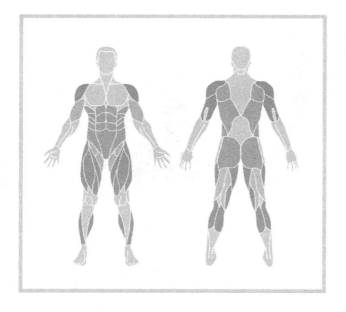

Difficulty

Sweat Inc.

DAREBEE HIIT WORKOUT © darebee.com

Level I 3 sets **Level II** 5 sets **Level III** 7 sets | 2 minutes rest

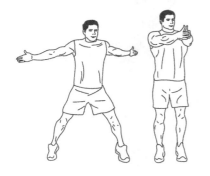

20sec seal jacks

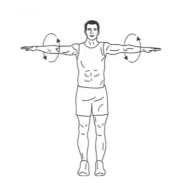

20sec raised arm circles

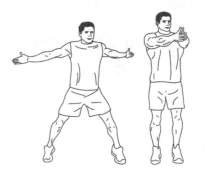

20sec seal jacks

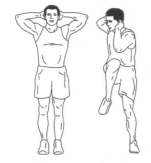

20sec knee-to-elbow

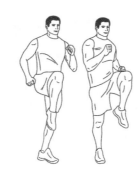

20sec high knees

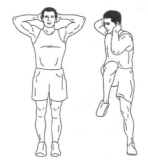

20sec knee-to-elbow

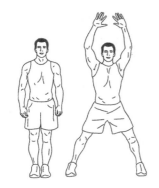

20sec jumping jacks

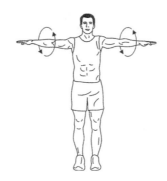

20sec raised arm circles

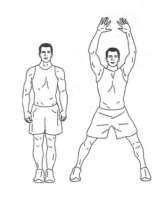

20sec jumping jacks

100 Toaster

Hunting Cylons means you need to be a machine yourself. This is a workout to help you build lower body strength and endurance. And don't forget that "burpees are everyone's favorite exercise" (said no one, ever).

Extra Credit: 30 seconds rest between sets.

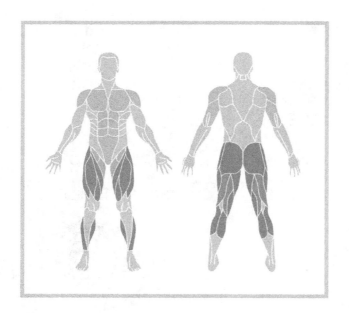

Difficulty

TOASTER

DAREBEE HIIT WORKOUT © darebee.com

Level I 3 sets **Level II** 5 sets **Level III** 7 sets | 2 minutes rest

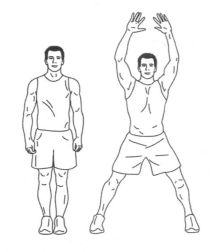

20sec jumping jacks

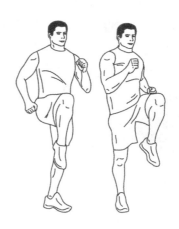

20sec high knees

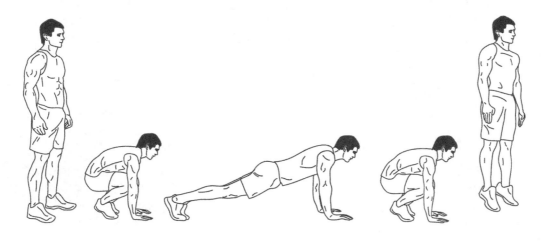

20sec basic burpees

Thank you!

Thank you for purchasing **100 No-Equipment Workouts Vol. 3**, DAREBEE project print edition. DAREBEE is a non-profit global fitness resource dedicated to making fitness accessible for everyone, no matter their circumstances. The project is supported exclusively via user donations and paperback royalties.

After printing costs and store fees every book developed by the DAREBEE project makes $1 and it goes directly into our project maintenance and development fund.

Each sale helps us keep the DAREBEE resource growing, maintain it and keep it up. Thank you for making a difference in its future!

Other books in this series include:

100 No-Equipment Workouts Vol 1.
100 No-Equipment Workouts Vol 2.
100 No-Equipment Workouts Vol 3.
100 Office Workouts
Pocket Workouts: 100 no-equipment workouts
ABS 100 Workouts: Visual Easy-To-Follow ABS Exercise Routines for All Fitness Levels

CPSIA information can be obtained
at www.ICGtesting.com
Printed in the USA
LVHW060248161119
637540LV00003B/16/P